Table of Content

Chapter 1: A Seed of Doubt

1.1 The Conventional Approach

In the heart of Metropolis, the bustling metropolis that never seemed to sleep, Dr. Sarah Wells found herself increasingly disillusioned with the conventional medical approach to treating hypothyroidism. As a passionate naturopath, she had witnessed firsthand the limitations of synthetic medications and the frustration of countless patients who struggled to find lasting relief from their debilitating symptoms.

The standard protocol was to prescribe synthetic thyroid hormones, often at a one-size-fits-all dosage, with the expectation that this would alleviate the patient's fatigue, weight gain, depression, and other manifestations of an underactive thyroid. However, time and again, Dr. Wells encountered individuals who remained trapped in a cycle of discomfort, their lives diminished by the persistent effects of this pervasive condition.

She couldn't help but question the wisdom of treating such a complex disorder with a simplistic, one-dimensional approach. Didn't the human body deserve a more nuanced, holistic understanding? Weren't there natural remedies, rooted in the ancient wisdom of traditional healing practices, that could offer a gentler, more comprehensive solution?

As she sat in her office, surrounded by the sterile white walls and the faint scent of disinfectant, Dr. Wells felt a growing unease. The conventional medical establishment had become so entrenched in its ways, so reliant on pharmaceutical interventions, that it seemed to have lost sight of the body's inherent ability to heal itself when provided with the right tools and guidance.

She knew she couldn't continue down this path, blindly subscribing to a system that too often failed to address the root causes of her patients' ailments. It was time to explore alternative approaches, to rediscover the ancient wisdom of natural healing, and to forge a new path that would empower individuals to reclaim their vitality and well-being.

With a renewed sense of determination, Dr. Wells began to question the status quo, challenging the assumptions that had long been ingrained in her medical training. She was ready to embark on a journey of discovery, one that would lead her to the very heart of holistic wellness and the transformative power of nature's thyroid solution.

1.2 Unraveling the Mystery

As Dr. Sarah Wells delved deeper into the realm of hypothyroidism, she found herself increasingly perplexed by the complexity of this often misunderstood condition. The conventional medical approach seemed to oversimplify the issue, treating it as a mere hormonal imbalance that could be addressed with synthetic thyroid replacement therapy.

However, the more she studied the intricate workings of the thyroid gland and its far-reaching impact on the body, the more she realized that this condition was a tangled web of interconnected factors, each influencing the other in ways that defied a one-size-fits-all solution.

Through her extensive research, Dr. Wells uncovered a multitude of potential contributors to hypothyroidism, ranging from environmental toxins and nutrient deficiencies to chronic stress and autoimmune disorders. She discovered that the thyroid, a small butterfly-shaped gland nestled at the base of the neck, was exquisitely sensitive to these external and internal influences, its delicate balance easily disrupted by the modern world's relentless assault.

As she pored over scientific studies and consulted with experts in various fields, a startling pattern began to emerge. Many of the factors implicated in hypothyroidism were inextricably linked to the way people lived their lives – the foods they consumed, the products they used, and the stresses they endured on a daily basis.

It became evident that the conventional approach, which focused solely on hormone replacement, was akin to treating a mere symptom while ignoring the underlying causes. Dr. Wells realized that true healing could only be achieved by addressing the root issues, by empowering individuals to make lifestyle changes that would support and nurture their thyroid function.

With each new insight, her determination grew stronger. She knew she had stumbled upon a critical piece of the puzzle, a missing link that could potentially unlock a world of healing for those suffering from hypothyroidism. The conventional medical establishment might be content with band-aid solutions, but Dr. Wells was driven by a deeper purpose – to unravel the mysteries of this condition and offer her patients a truly holistic path to wellness.

As she continued her quest, Dr. Wells found herself drawn to the ancient teachings of traditional healing modalities, each offering its own unique perspective on the intricate dance between the thyroid and the body's delicate equilibrium. She immersed herself in the study of herbal medicine, acupuncture, and mind-body practices, seeking to understand how these time-honored approaches could complement and enhance the conventional treatments.

It was a daunting task, but Dr. Wells was fueled by a burning desire to help her patients reclaim their vitality and break free from the shackles of hypothyroidism. With each step, she peeled back another layer of the mystery, inching closer to a holistic understanding that would revolutionize the way this condition was perceived and treated.

1.3 A Personal Revelation

As Dr. Sarah Wells delved deeper into her research, she couldn't help but reflect on her own personal journey with hypothyroidism. It was a condition that had plagued her family for generations, a silent burden passed down from mother to daughter, often misunderstood and mismanaged.

She vividly remembered her grandmother, a once vibrant and energetic woman, slowly succumbing to the debilitating effects of an underactive thyroid. Despite being prescribed synthetic hormones, her grandmother's health continued to deteriorate, her once radiant smile replaced by a permanent state of fatigue and brain fog.

Dr. Wells had been too young then to fully comprehend the complexities of the situation, but she could still recall the helplessness she felt as she witnessed her grandmother's struggle. It was a memory that had stayed with her, a constant reminder of the limitations of conventional medicine in addressing such a multifaceted condition.

As she grew older and embarked on her own medical journey, Dr. Wells found herself confronting the same challenges her grandmother had faced. Despite following the standard treatment protocols, she continued to experience lingering symptoms – persistent fatigue, stubborn weight gain, and bouts of depression that seemed to defy explanation.

It was a frustrating and disheartening experience, one that left her questioning the very foundations of her medical training. How could it be that modern medicine, with all its advancements and technological marvels, still struggled to effectively treat such a common condition?

The more she explored the conventional approach to hypothyroidism, the more she realized that it was a deeply flawed system, one that treated patients as mere statistics rather than unique individuals with complex biologies and life stories. It was a one-size-fits-all mentality that failed to account for the intricate interplay of genetics, environment, and lifestyle factors that contributed to the development and progression of the condition.

It was during this period of personal struggle and self-reflection that Dr. Wells experienced a profound revelation – a realization that would forever alter the course of her professional journey. She understood that true healing could only be achieved by embracing a holistic perspective, one that recognized the interconnectedness of mind, body, and spirit.

With a newfound determination, she began to explore alternative healing modalities, seeking wisdom from ancient traditions and modern scientific research alike. She immersed herself in the study of herbal medicine, delving into the vast pharmacopeia of nature's bounty and uncovering centuries-old remedies that had been overlooked by mainstream medicine.

She also discovered the profound impact of diet and lifestyle on thyroid function, learning how the foods we consume, the toxins we're exposed to, and the stresses we endure can all contribute to the development and exacerbation of hypothyroidism.

As she integrated these diverse perspectives, a new approach began to take shape – one that combined the best of conventional and complementary therapies, tailored to the unique needs of each individual patient. It was a holistic approach that empowered individuals to take an active role in their own healing journey, recognizing that true wellness extended far beyond the mere absence of disease.

For Dr. Wells, this personal revelation was a turning point, a moment of clarity that would shape the trajectory of her career and her mission to revolutionize the way hypothyroidism was understood and treated. It was a journey that would take her to the farthest corners of the world, seeking wisdom from traditional healers and exploring the healing power of nature's thyroid solution.

1.4 Challenging the Norm

As Dr. Sarah Wells delved deeper into her exploration of natural remedies for hypothyroidism, she found herself increasingly at odds with the prevailing medical establishment. The conventional approach, which relied heavily on synthetic hormone replacement therapy, had become so deeply entrenched that any deviation from the norm was met with skepticism and resistance.

Dr. Wells understood the weight of her actions – she was challenging long-held beliefs and practices that had been ingrained in medical professionals for decades. It was a daunting prospect, one that would require an unwavering commitment to her principles and a willingness to confront the very system she had been trained to uphold.

Yet, she could not ignore the mounting evidence that supported a more holistic approach to thyroid health. Through her research, she had uncovered a wealth of ancient wisdom and modern scientific findings that pointed to the efficacy of natural remedies, dietary modifications, and lifestyle interventions in addressing the root causes of hypothyroidism.

As she began to incorporate these alternative therapies into her practice, she witnessed firsthand the remarkable transformations her patients experienced. Individuals who had been trapped in a cycle of fatigue, weight gain, and emotional turmoil slowly regained their vitality, shedding excess pounds and rediscovering a sense of emotional equilibrium.

With each success story, Dr. Wells's conviction grew stronger. She could no longer turn a blind eye to the limitations of conventional medicine, nor could she ignore the profound healing potential of nature's thyroid solution.

However, her newfound approach was not without its critics. Some members of the medical community viewed her methods as unconventional and unproven, dismissing the centuries-old wisdom of traditional healing practices as mere pseudoscience. They questioned her credentials and her motives, accusing her of peddling false hope and endangering the health of her patients.

But Dr. Wells was undeterred. She understood that true progress often came at the cost of resistance, and she was prepared to weather the storm of skepticism and criticism. Armed with a deep well of knowledge and a steadfast belief in the power of holistic healing, she continued to refine her approach, tailoring each treatment plan to the unique needs of her patients.

In her clinic, she created a sanctuary where individuals could explore the transformative potential of natural remedies in a supportive and nurturing environment. She cultivated a team of like-minded professionals, including herbalists, acupuncturists, and nutritionists, who shared her vision of integrative care.

Together, they embarked on a journey of discovery, constantly expanding their understanding of the intricate interplay between the thyroid and the body's delicate balance. They studied ancient texts, explored new avenues of research, and collaborated with traditional healers from around the world, each encounter yielding new insights and deepening their commitment to this holistic approach.

As word of her success began to spread, Dr. Wells's clinic attracted a growing number of patients from far and wide, each seeking a path to healing that had eluded them through conventional means. With each new case, she gained invaluable experience and further refined her methods, constantly adapting and evolving to meet the unique needs of her diverse patient population.

Through it all, she remained steadfast in her conviction that challenging the norm was not an act of defiance, but rather a necessary step towards a more compassionate and effective approach to healthcare. By embracing the wisdom of ancient traditions and integrating it with modern scientific knowledge, she was paving the way for a new era of holistic wellness – one that recognized the intricate tapestry of mind, body, and spirit, and sought to nurture the body's innate ability to heal itself.

1.5 The Journey Begins

With a newfound sense of purpose and a burning desire to challenge the status quo, Dr. Sarah Wells embarked on a journey that would forever change the landscape of thyroid care. She knew that this path would be fraught with obstacles and skepticism, but her unwavering belief in the healing power of nature's thyroid solution fueled her determination.

The first step was to immerse herself in the ancient wisdom of traditional healing modalities. Dr. Wells spent countless hours poring over ancient texts, meticulously studying the teachings of Ayurvedic, Chinese, and indigenous healers who had long recognized the intricate connection between the thyroid and overall well-being.

She traveled to remote corners of the world, seeking out revered practitioners who had mastered the art of herbal medicine, acupuncture, and mind-body practices. With an open mind and a thirst for knowledge, she absorbed their teachings, learning to harness the potent properties of medicinal plants and the subtle energies that flow through the body's meridians.

Each encounter with these ancient traditions unveiled new layers of understanding, shedding light on the intricate interplay between the thyroid and the body's delicate equilibrium. Dr. Wells was humbled by the depth of wisdom contained within these time-honored practices, and she marveled at how modern medicine had overlooked such powerful healing modalities.

Armed with this newfound knowledge, she returned to her clinic with a renewed sense of purpose. She began to integrate these natural remedies and holistic approaches into her treatment plans, carefully tailoring each regimen to the unique needs of her patients.

For some, this meant incorporating herbal supplements and dietary modifications to support thyroid function and address nutrient deficiencies. For others, it involved exploring the therapeutic benefits of acupuncture, which could help restore the flow of vital energy and alleviate the physical and emotional manifestations of hypothyroidism.

Dr. Wells also recognized the profound impact of stress on thyroid health and incorporated mind-body practices such as meditation, yoga, and breathwork into her patients' care plans. She understood that true healing required a holistic approach that addressed not only the physical aspects of the condition but also the emotional and spiritual components.

As her patients began to experience the transformative effects of these natural therapies, word of Dr. Wells's innovative approach spread like wildfire. People from all walks of life, many of whom had been failed by conventional medicine, sought her out, desperate for a solution that could restore their vitality and reclaim their lives.

With each success story, Dr. Wells's confidence in her methods grew stronger. She witnessed firsthand the profound changes that occurred when individuals embraced a holistic approach to thyroid health. Fatigue gave way to renewed energy, stubborn weight melted away, and emotional turmoil was replaced by a sense of peace and clarity.

Yet, even as her clinic flourished and her reputation grew, Dr. Wells remained grounded in her mission. She knew that true change would require more than just individual healing – it would demand a paradigm shift in the way society approached thyroid care and, indeed, healthcare as a whole.

Undeterred by the skepticism and resistance from the medical establishment, Dr. Wells began to share her knowledge and insights with a wider audience. She published articles, gave lectures, and hosted workshops, spreading the message of nature's thyroid solution and the transformative power of holistic healing.

With each encounter, she inspired others to question the status quo and explore alternative paths to wellness. Her passion was contagious, and soon, a grassroots movement began to take shape, with individuals from all walks of life embracing the principles of integrative care and demanding a more comprehensive approach to thyroid health.

As the journey continued, Dr. Wells faced countless challenges and setbacks, but her unwavering determination and her deep-seated belief in the healing potential of nature's thyroid solution kept her moving forward. She knew that this was more than just a personal quest – it was a mission to revolutionize the way society approached health and wellness, one step at a time.

Chapter 2: Voices from the Shadows

2.1 Fatigue's Embrace

In the heart of Metropolis, an invisible epidemic was silently unfolding, its insidious tendrils reaching into the lives of countless individuals, robbing them of their vitality and diminishing the very essence of their being. This affliction was not a contagious disease or a visible ailment; rather, it was a pervasive state of exhaustion that permeated every aspect of their existence.

For Sarah Henderson, the relentless fatigue was a constant companion, its weight bearing down upon her like an invisible cloak. Each morning, she would awake feeling as though she had never slept, her muscles aching and her mind shrouded in a thick fog of lethargy. Even the simplest tasks, such as getting dressed or preparing a meal, became monumental challenges that sapped her of what little energy she had.

Yet, Sarah's story was not unique. Across the city, individuals from all walks of life found themselves trapped in a similar cycle of exhaustion, their once vibrant lives reduced to a mere shadow of their former selves.

Michael, a successful corporate executive, found himself nodding off during important meetings, his once razor-sharp focus dulled by the overwhelming fatigue that consumed him. He would return home each evening, utterly drained, unable to engage with his family or pursue the hobbies that had once brought him joy.

For Emily, a young mother of two, the fatigue was a constant battle. She would drag herself through the day, struggling to keep up with the demands of her children and household, her once boundless energy replaced by a deep, bone-weary tiredness that seemed to seep into every fiber of her being.

These individuals, and countless others like them, had become unwitting victims of hypothyroidism – a condition that had long been misunderstood and often dismissed as a mere inconvenience. Yet, for those caught in its grip, the impact was profound, reaching far beyond the realm of physical discomfort and casting a pall over every aspect of their lives.

The fatigue was not a fleeting sensation, but rather a persistent, all-consuming force that sapped their motivation, their productivity, and their very sense of self. It was a silent thief, stealing away the precious moments and experiences that should have been filled with joy and fulfillment.

Worse still, many of these individuals had sought help from the conventional medical establishment, only to be met with dismissive attitudes or ineffective treatments. Their concerns were often minimized, their symptoms dismissed as mere side effects of aging or the stresses of modern life.

But for those trapped in fatigue's embrace, there was no solace in such platitudes. They longed for a deeper understanding, a compassionate approach that recognized the profound impact this condition had on their lives and offered a path towards true healing and restoration.

It was in this climate of frustration and despair that Dr. Sarah Wells emerged as a beacon of hope. Her holistic approach to thyroid care resonated with those who had lost faith in the conventional medical system, offering them a glimmer of possibility – a chance to reclaim the energy and vitality that had been stolen from them.

As word of her innovative methods spread, more and more individuals sought her out, eager to share their stories and find solace in a community that understood their struggles. In the safe haven of her clinic, these once-silenced voices found the courage to speak out, their tales of exhaustion and perseverance echoing through the halls and serving as a rallying cry for change.

2.2 Weight Woes

Alongside the relentless fatigue that plagued those suffering from hypothyroidism, another insidious symptom had taken hold – an unyielding struggle with weight gain. For many, this battle felt like a cruel betrayal of their own bodies, as if their very metabolism had turned against them, defying even the most stringent diets and exercise regimens.

Lisa, a fitness enthusiast who had always taken pride in her active lifestyle and toned physique, found herself utterly bewildered by the sudden and seemingly inexplicable weight gain. Despite adhering to her rigorous workout routine and meticulously tracking her caloric intake, the pounds continued to pile on, leaving her feeling defeated and dejected.

"I would look in the mirror and not recognize the person staring back at me," Lisa confided in Dr. Wells during one of their sessions. "It was like my body was sabotaging all my efforts, no matter how hard I tried."

Her story was echoed by countless others who had sought solace in Dr. Wells's integrative approach to thyroid care. Paul, a former athlete, had watched helplessly as his once-lean frame became obscured by layers of stubborn fat, no matter how strictly he followed his diet and exercise plan.

"I felt like a prisoner in my own body," he confessed, his voice laced with frustration. "It was as if someone had flipped a switch, and my metabolism just ground to a halt."

For these individuals, the weight gain was more than just a physical burden; it was a psychological and emotional weight that threatened to crush their self-confidence and sense of identity. They found themselves withdrawing from social situations, ashamed of their changing appearances and haunted by the constant fear of judgment from others.

Worse still, their struggles were often dismissed or trivialized by those around them, who offered well-meaning but ultimately misguided advice about portion control and willpower. These individuals felt isolated and misunderstood, their experiences invalidated by a society that placed undue emphasis on outward appearances and quick-fix solutions.

It was a vicious cycle – the weight gain fueled feelings of low self-worth and depression, which in turn exacerbated the metabolic imbalances that contributed to the condition. Many found themselves caught in a downward spiral, their once-vibrant lives reduced to a constant battle against the scale and the relentless pursuit of a seemingly unattainable goal.

But in the sanctuary of Dr. Wells's clinic, these individuals found a safe haven where their struggles were not only acknowledged but also understood on a profound level. Here, they discovered a community of like-minded individuals who had walked the same path, each with their own stories of frustration and perseverance.

Through Dr. Wells's holistic approach, which combined dietary modifications, herbal supplements, and stress-management techniques, these individuals began to experience glimmers of hope. Slowly but surely, their bodies began to respond, and the stubborn weight that had once seemed immovable started to melt away.

For some, it was a gradual process, with incremental changes that built upon one another, while for others, the transformation was more dramatic, as if a switch had been flipped, reigniting their metabolism and restoring their vitality.

Regardless of the pace, each victory was celebrated as a hard-won triumph, a testament to the power of perseverance and the efficacy of Dr. Wells's integrative methods. As these individuals reclaimed their physical health and self-confidence, they also experienced a profound shift in their emotional and psychological well-being, shedding the weight of shame and stigma that had burdened them for so long.

In the halls of Dr. Wells's clinic, the echoes of their struggles and triumphs resonated, serving as a rallying cry for a more compassionate and effective approach to thyroid care – one that recognized the intricate interplay between physical, emotional, and spiritual well-being, and empowered individuals to reclaim their vitality and embrace their true selves.

2.3 Emotional Turmoil

While the physical manifestations of hypothyroidism, such as fatigue and weight gain, were often the most visible and widely discussed symptoms, there was another insidious aspect of this condition that lingered in the shadows – the emotional turmoil that threatened to consume those in its grip.

For many, the emotional toll of hypothyroidism was a silent battle waged within the confines of their own minds, a struggle that often went unnoticed and misunderstood by those around them. It was a cyclone of emotions that could strike without warning, leaving them feeling overwhelmed, isolated, and utterly adrift in a sea of despair.

Sarah, a once-vibrant young woman who had always been the life of the party, found herself withdrawing from social situations as the emotional weight of her condition grew heavier. What had once been a bubbling well of confidence and joy had been replaced by a profound sense of melancholy that seemed to permeate every aspect of her life.

"It was like a dark cloud had descended upon me," she confided in Dr. Wells during one of their sessions. "No matter how hard I tried to shake it off, the sadness just lingered, seeping into every moment and tainting even the most joyous of occasions."

For others, the emotional turmoil manifested as a pervasive sense of anxiety and uncertainty, a constant state of unease that left them feeling on edge and unable to fully relax. Emily, a successful marketing executive, found herself plagued by racing thoughts and irrational fears that seemed to consume her waking hours.

"I would lie awake at night, my mind spinning with worries and doubts," she shared with Dr. Wells. "It was like a constant state of fight-or-flight, even though there was no real threat. I felt like I was losing control of my own thoughts and emotions."

The emotional toll of hypothyroidism was not limited to sadness or anxiety alone; for some, it was a volatile cocktail of conflicting emotions that left them feeling utterly unmoored and adrift. One day, they might find themselves consumed by overwhelming anger and irritability, lashing out at loved ones for seemingly innocuous transgressions. The next, they might be plunged into the depths of despair, unable to find joy or meaning in even the simplest of pleasures.

This emotional rollercoaster was not only exhausting but also profoundly isolating. Those around them struggled to understand the depths of their turmoil, often attributing their emotional upheaval to stress, hormones, or even personal failings. This lack of understanding only served to deepen the sense of isolation and despair, creating a vicious cycle that threatened to consume them entirely.

It was in the safe haven of Dr. Wells's clinic that these individuals found solace and understanding. Here, they discovered a community of like-minded souls who had walked the same path, each with their own stories of emotional struggle and resilience.

Through her holistic approach, which incorporated not only dietary and lifestyle modifications but also mind-body practices such as meditation and counseling, Dr. Wells sought to address the emotional toll of hypothyroidism head-on. She recognized that true healing could not be achieved by simply addressing the physical symptoms alone; rather, it required a deep understanding of the intricate interplay between the mind, body, and spirit.

Slowly but surely, those who had once felt lost in the depths of emotional turmoil began to find their way back to a sense of equilibrium. The dark clouds of despair began to dissipate, replaced by glimmers of hope and moments of clarity. The constant state of anxiety and unease gradually gave way to a newfound sense of calm and inner peace.

For some, the journey was a winding path, with both triumphs and setbacks along the way. But within the walls of Dr. Wells's clinic, they found solace in the shared experience, drawing strength from one another's stories and the unwavering belief that healing was not only possible but attainable.

As they emerged from the shadows of emotional turmoil, these individuals rediscovered the joy and vibrancy that had once been integral to their lives. They found themselves laughing more freely, embracing new experiences, and rekindling the connections that had once been strained by the weight of their emotional burdens.

In the halls of Dr. Wells's clinic, the echoes of their journeys resonated, serving as a powerful testimony to the transformative power of holistic healing and the indomitable strength of the human spirit. It was a reminder that even in the darkest of times, hope could be found – a beacon of light that would guide them towards a path of emotional well-being and a renewed sense of wholeness.

2.4 The Unspoken Struggle

Amidst the myriad of physical and emotional challenges posed by hypothyroidism, there existed an often-overlooked aspect of this condition – the silent, unspoken struggles that threatened to undermine the very fabric of personal relationships and social connections.

For many individuals grappling with the effects of an underactive thyroid, the strain on their personal and professional lives was palpable, yet rarely acknowledged or understood by those around them. It was a silent battle waged within the confines of their own homes and workplaces, a constant effort to maintain a semblance of normalcy while silently suffering from the debilitating symptoms that robbed them of their vitality and well-being.

Rachel, a devoted mother of three, found herself struggling to keep up with the demands of her family and household duties. Once a source of unwavering energy and joy, she now found herself utterly drained, unable to muster the enthusiasm and patience required to be the parent she aspired to be.

"I would look at my children and feel overwhelming guilt," she confided in Dr. Wells, her voice trembling with emotion. "They deserved a mother who was present and engaged, but instead, they had to contend with a shell of a person, someone who was constantly fatigued and emotionally detached."

For Michael, a rising star in the corporate world, the unspoken struggle manifested in the form of professional setbacks and strained relationships with colleagues. His once-sharp focus and productivity had been replaced by a fog of exhaustion and forgetfulness, leading to missed deadlines and crucial mistakes that threatened to derail his promising career.

"It was like I was constantly swimming against the current, trying to keep my head above water while everyone around me seemed to be effortlessly gliding through their work," he shared with Dr. Wells. "I felt like a failure, unable to live up to the expectations that had been set for me."

The strain on personal and professional relationships was not solely rooted in physical or cognitive limitations; for many, the emotional turmoil that accompanied hypothyroidism played a significant role in fracturing once-strong bonds. Mood swings, irritability, and emotional detachment often led to misunderstandings, conflicts, and a growing sense of isolation within their own circles.

Emily, a once-vibrant social butterfly, found herself withdrawing from her friends and loved ones, unable to muster the energy or emotional bandwidth required to maintain those cherished connections.

"It was like I was slowly slipping away from the person I once was," she confessed to Dr. Wells. "My friends couldn't understand why I was constantly canceling plans or why I seemed so distant and withdrawn. They couldn't see the invisible weight that was dragging me down, the constant struggle to simply exist in the world."

For these individuals, the unspoken struggle was a silent burden that weighed heavily upon their shoulders, threatening to erode the very foundations of their personal and professional lives. They found themselves trapped in a cycle of misunderstanding and guilt, their loved ones and colleagues unable to comprehend the depths of their suffering.

It was in the safe haven of Dr. Wells's clinic that these unspoken struggles found a voice – a sanctuary where they could openly share their experiences without fear of judgment or dismissal. Here, they discovered a community of like-minded individuals who had walked the same path, each with their own tales of personal and professional strife.

Through her holistic approach, which recognized the intricate interplay between physical, emotional, and social well-being, Dr. Wells sought to address the often-overlooked impact of hypothyroidism on personal relationships and professional endeavors. She encouraged open communication, fostering a supportive environment where loved ones and colleagues could gain a deeper understanding of the challenges faced by those afflicted with this condition.

Slowly but surely, as these individuals began to reclaim their vitality and regain a sense of emotional balance, the strain on their personal and professional lives began to ease. Connections that had once been frayed were mended, and misunderstandings gave way to newfound empathy and understanding.

For some, the journey involved difficult conversations and the acknowledgment of past mistakes or missteps. For others, it was a process of rediscovering the joy and fulfillment that had once been integral to their personal and professional pursuits.

Within the walls of Dr. Wells's clinic, the echoes of these unspoken struggles resonated, serving as a powerful reminder of the far-reaching impact of hypothyroidism and the importance of a holistic, compassionate approach to healing. It was a testament to the resilience of the human spirit and the transformative power of understanding and support.

As these individuals emerged from the shadows of their unspoken battles, they found themselves embracing a newfound sense of connection and purpose – a renewed appreciation for the richness of personal relationships and the fulfillment that comes from pursuing one's passions and professional goals with vigor and vitality.

2.5 A Shared Burden

Amid the myriad of challenges and struggles that accompanied hypothyroidism, a profound sense of isolation often took root, casting a pall over the lives of those afflicted. However, within the sanctuary of Dr. Wells's clinic, a powerful revelation emerged – the realization that they were not alone in their battles, but rather part of a vast community united by a shared experience.

As individuals from all walks of life converged, each carrying their own unique stories and burdens, a tapestry of shared understanding began to unfold. The once-lonely journeys of fatigue, weight woes, emotional turmoil, and unspoken struggles suddenly found resonance in the experiences of others, creating a powerful sense of kinship and validation.

For Sarah, a young professional who had long felt misunderstood and dismissed by those around her, the discovery of this community was nothing short of life-changing. "When I first walked through those doors, I felt like I was carrying the weight of the world on my shoulders," she confided to Dr. Wells. "But then I heard the stories of others, and I realized that I wasn't alone in this fight. It was like a veil had been lifted, and I could finally breathe again."

This shared understanding extended beyond the physical symptoms and emotional challenges of hypothyroidism; it also encompassed the unspoken struggles that had long remained hidden from view. The strain on personal relationships, the professional setbacks, and the overwhelming sense of guilt and self-doubt that had plagued so many found solace in the collective experiences of this tight-knit community.

"For years, I thought I was the only one going through this," confessed Michael, a once-successful businessman whose career had been derailed by the relentless grip of hypothyroidism. "But here, I found others who understood the toll it took on our professional lives, the constant battle to stay afloat while struggling with exhaustion and mental fog."

Within the walls of Dr. Wells's clinic, these individuals found a safe haven where they could openly share their stories without fear of judgment or dismissal. Together, they formed a powerful support network, offering encouragement, empathy, and practical advice born from lived experiences.

For some, the simple act of being heard and understood was a profound source of healing, a balm for the wounds inflicted by years of isolation and misunderstanding. As they shared their journeys, they found solace in the knowledge that they were not alone, that their struggles were valid and deserving of compassion.

But the power of this shared community extended far beyond emotional support alone. It also served as a wellspring of knowledge and inspiration, as individuals exchanged insights, strategies, and hard-won wisdom that had helped them navigate the challenges of hypothyroidism.

"When I first started incorporating the dietary changes and lifestyle modifications that Dr. Wells recommended, it felt like an uphill battle," recalled Emily, a young mother who had once struggled with debilitating fatigue and weight gain. "But then I connected with others who had been through the same journey, and they shared their tips and tricks – little things that made a world of difference in my healing process."

As these individuals celebrated each other's triumphs and offered solace during setbacks, a powerful bond was forged – a bond that transcended age, background, or social status. They were united by a common goal: to reclaim their vitality, restore their sense of well-being, and emerge from the shadows of hypothyroidism as stronger, more resilient versions of themselves.

In the halls of Dr. Wells's clinic, the echoes of their shared stories resonated, creating a symphony of hope and perseverance. It was a constant reminder that even in the darkest of times, they were never truly alone – that there was strength in numbers and power in the collective wisdom of a community that understood the depths of their struggles.

As they embarked on their individual journeys towards healing and wholeness, these individuals carried with them the knowledge that they were part of something greater – a movement towards a more compassionate and holistic approach to healthcare, one that recognized the profound interconnectedness of mind, body, and spirit.

And in that shared understanding, they found the courage and resilience to forge ahead, secure in the knowledge that their burdens were no longer theirs alone to bear, but rather a collective weight distributed among a community of kindred spirits, united in their pursuit of a brighter, more vibrant future.

Chapter 3: The Wisdom of Ancients

3.1 Unlocking Ancient Texts

In her quest to unravel the mysteries of hypothyroidism and unlock the healing potential of nature's thyroid solution, Dr. Sarah Wells found herself drawn to the ancient wisdom that had been preserved through the ages. It was a journey that would take her far beyond the confines of modern medicine, delving into the rich tapestry of traditional healing modalities that had been woven by cultures across the globe.

Her first stop was the vast repository of ancient texts that had been meticulously curated by scholars and healers throughout history. Here, amidst the musty scent of aged parchment and the whispers of forgotten tongues, Dr. Wells discovered a world of knowledge that had long been overlooked by the conventional medical establishment.

She pored over the yellowed pages of Ayurvedic texts, marveling at the intricate understanding of the body's delicate balance and the role of the thyroid in maintaining overall well-being. The ancient Indian practitioners had recognized the interconnectedness of mind, body, and spirit, and their teachings offered a holistic perspective on thyroid health that resonated deeply with Dr. Wells.

Next, she immersed herself in the ancient Chinese medical texts, tracing the intricate pathways of energy flow and the profound impact of the thyroid on this life-sustaining current. She was captivated by the intricate descriptions of the meridian system and the delicate dance of yin and yang, which governed the body's hormonal equilibrium.

As she delved deeper into these ancient texts, Dr. Wells found herself transported to a realm where the boundaries between science and spirituality blurred, where the human body was revered as a sacred vessel, and the art of healing was elevated to a sacred practice.

In the weathered pages of indigenous healing traditions, she uncovered a wealth of knowledge that had been passed down through generations, each page imbued with the wisdom of those who had come before. From the potent herbal remedies of the Amazonian rainforest to the ancient rituals of the Native American tribes, Dr. Wells was humbled by the depth of understanding these cultures possessed regarding the thyroid's intricate workings.

With each turn of the page, she felt a growing sense of awe and reverence for the ancient healers who had walked this path centuries before her. Their insights, born from a deep connection to the natural world and a profound respect for the body's inherent wisdom, offered a stark contrast to the often-reductionist approach of modern medicine.

Yet, Dr. Wells was not content to merely study these ancient texts as relics of a bygone era. Instead, she sought to unlock the practical applications of their teachings, to bridge the chasm between the ancient and the modern, and to integrate these time-honored wisdom into her holistic approach to thyroid care.

She spent countless hours cross-referencing the ancient texts with the latest scientific research, searching for points of convergence and validation. To her astonishment, she found that many of the principles espoused by these ancient traditions were being substantiated by cutting-edge studies in fields such as epigenetics, nutritional biochemistry, and mind-body medicine.

Armed with this newfound understanding, Dr. Wells began to weave the threads of ancient wisdom and modern science into a tapestry of knowledge that would form the foundation of her integrative approach to thyroid health. She synthesized the dietary recommendations of Ayurveda with the latest nutritional insights, incorporating the healing properties of herbs and spices that had been revered for millennia.

From the Chinese medical texts, she learned to harness the power of acupuncture and energy-balancing techniques, integrating them seamlessly with conventional therapies to restore the body's delicate hormonal equilibrium.

And from the indigenous healing traditions, she gleaned a profound respect for the interconnectedness of all living beings, recognizing that true healing could only be achieved by nurturing a harmonious relationship between the human body and the natural world.

As she wove these ancient and modern strands together, a new paradigm of thyroid care began to take shape – one that honored the wisdom of the ancients while embracing the cutting-edge advancements of modern science. It was a holistic approach that recognized the intricate tapestry of physical, emotional, and spiritual well-being, and sought to nurture the body's innate ability to heal itself.

Through her tireless efforts and unwavering dedication, Dr. Wells had unlocked the ancient secrets that had been hidden within the musty pages of long-forgotten texts, breathing new life into these timeless teachings and ushering in a renaissance of holistic thyroid care.

3.2 Forgotten Healing Arts

As Dr. Sarah Wells delved deeper into the ancient wisdom of traditional healing modalities, she found herself drawn to the forgotten healing arts that had once flourished across diverse cultures and civilizations. These time-honored practices, though often dismissed or overlooked by modern medicine, held within them a profound understanding of the body's intricate workings and a reverence for the healing power of nature.

One such art that captured Dr. Wells's attention was the ancient practice of energy healing, which had its roots in the Eastern philosophies of Qi and Prana. She marveled at the way these ancient traditions viewed the human body as a conduit for life-sustaining energy, with the thyroid gland playing a pivotal role in regulating and harmonizing this flow.

Through her studies, she learned of the intricate meridian system that ran like invisible rivers throughout the body, carrying this vital energy to every cell and organ. When these pathways became blocked or imbalanced, the teachings held, disease and disharmony would inevitably follow.

Intrigued by these ancient concepts, Dr. Wells sought out revered masters of energy healing practices, such as Reiki, Qigong, and acupuncture. She immersed herself in their teachings, learning to perceive and manipulate the subtle energies that flowed through the body with a deft touch and a singular focus.

As she witnessed the profound impact these practices had on her patients, Dr. Wells couldn't help but marvel at the ingenuity and wisdom of these ancient healers. They had developed intricate systems for restoring balance and harmony to the body's energy flow, all without the aid of modern technology or pharmaceutical interventions.

Another forgotten healing art that captivated Dr. Wells was the ancient practice of plant medicine, which had been revered by countless indigenous cultures throughout history. She was awed by the intricate knowledge these communities possessed regarding the healing properties of plants and their ability to harness nature's bounty for the benefit of human health.

From the lush rainforests of the Amazon to the arid deserts of the Middle East, Dr. Wells sought out revered herbalists and shamans, learning the intricate art of plant identification, preparation, and application. She marveled at the depth of understanding these practitioners possessed, having developed an intimate relationship with the natural world through generations of observation and experimentation.

As she studied the ancient texts and engaged in hands-on learning, Dr. Wells discovered a wealth of plant-based remedies that had the potential to support thyroid health and alleviate the debilitating symptoms of hypothyroidism. From adaptogenic herbs that helped the body cope with stress to nutrient-dense superfoods that nourished the gland, she was amazed by the sheer diversity and potency of nature's pharmacopeia.

Yet, in her pursuit of these forgotten healing arts, Dr. Wells encountered more than just practical knowledge and therapeutic modalities. She found herself immersed in a profound reverence for the natural world and a deep respect for the interconnectedness of all living beings.

These ancient traditions taught her to view the human body not as a collection of isolated parts, but rather as a microcosm of the larger ecosystem, intricately woven into the fabric of the natural world. They emphasized the importance of living in harmony with the cycles of nature, honoring the rhythms of the seasons, and nourishing the body with the bounty of the earth.

As she integrated these ancient principles into her holistic approach to thyroid care, Dr. Wells witnessed remarkable transformations in her patients. Not only did they experience relief from their physical symptoms, but they also cultivated a deeper sense of connection to the natural world, a renewed appreciation for the healing power of plants, and a greater understanding of the delicate balance that governs all life.

Through her dedication to uncovering and preserving these forgotten healing arts, Dr. Wells had become a torchbearer for a renaissance of holistic wellness – a movement that sought to rekindle the ancient wisdom that had been obscured by the relentless march of modernity. In doing so, she was not only revolutionizing the way thyroid disorders were treated but also paving the way for a more harmonious and sustainable relationship between humanity and the natural world.

3.3 Nature's Bounty

In her quest to unlock the secrets of holistic thyroid healing, Dr. Sarah Wells found herself drawn deeper into the embrace of nature, marveling at the boundless bounty it offered for those willing to delve into its mysteries. As she explored the ancient wisdom of traditional healing practices, one recurring theme emerged – a profound reverence for the healing power of plants.

From the lush rainforests of the Amazon to the rugged mountain ranges of the Himalayas, Dr. Wells immersed herself in the study of ethnobotany, learning from revered healers and shamans who had cultivated an intimate relationship with the flora that surrounded them. She was humbled by the depth of their knowledge, which had been passed down through generations, each plant's properties and applications carefully documented and refined over centuries of observation and experimentation.

In the heart of the Amazonian jungle, she encountered a revered curandero, a master of plant medicine, who taught her the intricate art of identifying and preparing herbal remedies. With a deft hand and a keen eye, he guided her through the verdant foliage, introducing her to plants with names as exotic as their healing properties.

Dr. Wells marveled at the curandero's ability to discern the subtle nuances of each plant, from the distinct aroma of its leaves to the intricate patterns adorning its bark. It was as if he could converse with the very essence of nature itself, gleaning insights that would forever elude those who merely observed from afar.

Under his tutelage, she learned to prepare tinctures, decoctions, and infusions, each one a potent elixir distilled from the earth's botanical treasures. She was amazed at the potency of these natural remedies, many of which had been used for centuries to treat a wide array of ailments, including thyroid disorders.

From the adaptogenic properties of ashwagandha, which helped the body cope with stress and restore hormonal balance, to the nutrient-rich superfood maca, which nourished the thyroid gland with a bounty of essential minerals and compounds, Dr. Wells discovered a veritable pharmacopeia of plant-based allies in her quest for holistic healing.

As she ventured further afield, she encountered other indigenous communities who had cultivated their own unique traditions of plant medicine. In the arid deserts of the Middle East, she learned of the healing properties of herbs like black seed and fenugreek, which had been revered for their ability to support thyroid function and alleviate the symptoms of hypothyroidism.

In the rugged mountains of the Himalayas, she was introduced to the ancient art of Ayurvedic medicine, a holistic system that viewed the body as a delicate balance of three doshas, or humors. Here, she learned to harness the power of spices like turmeric and ginger, not only for their culinary delights but also for their potent anti-inflammatory and hormone-balancing properties.

With each encounter, Dr. Wells's respect for the healing power of plants grew deeper, as did her determination to integrate these natural remedies into her holistic approach to thyroid care. She marveled at the way these ancient traditions had preserved and cultivated knowledge that had been all but forgotten by modern medicine, which had become increasingly reliant on synthetic pharmaceuticals and reductionist interventions.

Yet, Dr. Wells's journey was not merely a quest for practical knowledge; it was a profound reconnection with the natural world and a deepening of her reverence for the intricate web of life that sustained all beings. As she immersed herself in these ancient traditions, she was reminded of the delicate balance that governs all ecosystems, and the vital role that plants play in maintaining that equilibrium.

Through her studies, she came to understand that true healing could not be achieved through isolated interventions or synthetic compounds alone. Rather, it required a holistic embrace of nature's bounty, a recognition of the intricate interplay between the human body and the vast tapestry of life that surrounded it.

With each plant she encountered, each remedy she prepared, and each indigenous tradition she explored, Dr. Wells felt herself becoming more attuned to the rhythms of the natural world. She learned to honor the cycles of the seasons, to respect the delicate balance of ecosystems, and to cultivate a deep appreciation for the gifts that the earth so generously bestowed upon those who walked its paths with reverence and humility.

In the verdant embrace of nature's bounty, Dr. Wells had found not only a wellspring of healing remedies but also a profound spiritual awakening – a realization that true wellness could only be achieved by reconnecting with the ancient wisdom that had guided humanity's relationship with the natural world for millennia.

3.4 Holistic Harmony

As Dr. Wells delved deeper into the ancient texts, a profound realization dawned upon her – the key to true healing lay in embracing a holistic approach that harmonized the body, mind, and spirit. This revelation shattered the conventional boundaries of medicine and opened her eyes to a world of possibilities.

In the dusty pages of ancient scrolls, she discovered intricate philosophies that viewed the human body as a microcosm of the universe, a delicate balance of energies and elements. The ancient sages believed that illness arose from an imbalance within this intricate system, and the path to wellness involved restoring harmony on all levels.

One such philosophy that resonated deeply with Dr. Wells was the ancient Chinese concept of Yin and Yang. This principle taught that all aspects of life, including health and disease, were governed by the dynamic interplay of opposing yet complementary forces. When Yin and Yang were in balance, the body thrived; when they fell out of sync, ailments manifested.

Intrigued by this holistic perspective, Dr. Wells immersed herself in the study of Traditional Chinese Medicine (TCM). She learned about the intricate network of meridians that carried life-giving energy, or Qi, throughout the body. Blockages or imbalances in this flow were believed to be the root cause of many ailments, including thyroid disorders.

As she explored the principles of TCM, Dr. Wells was struck by the emphasis placed on treating the whole person, not just the symptoms. The ancient healers recognized that physical ailments were often intertwined with emotional, mental, and spiritual imbalances, and true healing required addressing all aspects of an individual's well-being.

This holistic approach resonated deeply with Dr. Wells, as she had witnessed firsthand how stress, anxiety, and emotional turmoil could exacerbate the symptoms of hypothyroidism. She realized that her patients needed more than just a pill to manage their condition; they needed a comprehensive approach that addressed the underlying imbalances in their lives.

Inspired by these ancient teachings, Dr. Wells began to incorporate holistic practices into her treatment plans. She encouraged her patients to engage in gentle exercises like Tai Chi and Qigong, which were designed to promote the flow of Qi and cultivate a sense of inner peace. She also introduced them to the practice of meditation, which had been shown to reduce stress and promote emotional well-being.

As her patients embraced these holistic practices, Dr. Wells witnessed remarkable transformations. Patients who had previously struggled with fatigue and lethargy reported feeling more energized and vibrant. Those grappling with emotional turmoil found a sense of calm and clarity. Even physical symptoms like weight gain and hair loss began to improve as the body's natural balance was restored.

Dr. Wells was humbled by the profound impact of these ancient wisdom traditions and their ability to complement conventional medical treatments. She realized that true healing required a synergistic approach that addressed the multifaceted nature of human existence.

Inspired by this newfound understanding, Dr. Wells began to incorporate elements of other holistic traditions into her practice. She studied the principles of Ayurveda, the ancient Indian system of medicine that emphasized the importance of balance between the body's three doshas, or energies. She learned about the healing properties of herbs and spices, and how they could be used to support thyroid function and overall well-being.

Dr. Wells also explored the wisdom of indigenous cultures, whose deep connection to nature and respect for the earth's cycles offered valuable insights into the art of healing. She learned about the power of plant medicines, the significance of rituals and ceremonies, and the importance of honoring the interconnectedness of all living beings.

As she wove these diverse threads of wisdom into her practice, Dr. Wells witnessed a profound shift in her patients' journeys toward wellness. They began to embrace a more holistic lifestyle, one that honored the delicate balance between mind, body, and spirit. They learned to listen to the wisdom of their bodies, to nourish themselves with wholesome foods, and to cultivate a sense of inner peace and gratitude.

Through her exploration of ancient healing traditions, Dr. Wells had uncovered a path that transcended the limitations of conventional medicine. She had discovered a way to treat her patients as whole beings, addressing not just their physical ailments but also the emotional, mental, and spiritual aspects of their lives.

As she stood at the crossroads of ancient wisdom and modern science, Dr. Wells felt a deep sense of purpose and determination. She knew that her journey had only just begun, but she was committed to sharing the transformative power of holistic healing with the world, one patient at a time.

3.5 A Newfound Path

Dr. Wells stood in the tranquil garden, surrounded by a kaleidoscope of vibrant blooms and the soothing melodies of a trickling fountain. The ancient texts she had uncovered, coupled with the wisdom of holistic healers from around the world, had opened her eyes to a newfound path – one that harmonized the body, mind, and spirit in the pursuit of true wellness.

As she breathed in the fragrant air, a sense of clarity washed over her. The conventional approach to treating hypothyroidism, with its reliance on synthetic medications and disregard for the body's intricate balance, had left her disillusioned. But now, armed with the knowledge of nature's bounty and the timeless principles of holistic healing, she felt a renewed sense of purpose.

The journey had been arduous, filled with countless hours of research, consultations with experts, and a relentless pursuit of understanding. Yet, with each step, the pieces of the puzzle fell into place, revealing a tapestry of interconnected elements that held the key to restoring thyroid health.

One of the most profound revelations came from the ancient Ayurvedic texts, which emphasized the importance of balancing the doshas – the fundamental energies that govern the body's functions. By aligning these energies through dietary modifications, herbal remedies, and mindful practices, the body's innate healing mechanisms could be unleashed.

Dr. Wells recalled the words of a revered Ayurvedic practitioner she had met during her travels: "The thyroid is a delicate gland, easily disrupted by the imbalances of modern life. To restore its harmony, we must nourish the body, calm the mind, and nurture the spirit."

Those words resonated deeply within her, echoing the principles she had encountered in various healing traditions around the world. From the traditional Chinese medicine concept of chi, or vital life force, to the Native American belief in the interconnectedness of all living beings, a common thread emerged – the recognition that true healing transcends the physical realm and encompasses the entirety of one's being.

As she contemplated these insights, Dr. Wells felt a renewed sense of purpose. The path ahead would not be easy, for she would face resistance from those entrenched in the conventional medical paradigm. But she was determined to forge ahead, guided by the wisdom of the ancients and the unwavering belief that nature held the keys to unlocking the body's innate healing potential.

With a renewed sense of conviction, Dr. Wells began to outline her holistic approach to thyroid health. At its core would be a comprehensive treatment plan that addressed the root causes of hypothyroidism, rather than merely masking the symptoms.

Dietary modifications would play a crucial role, emphasizing the consumption of nutrient-dense, whole foods that nourished the thyroid and supported overall metabolic function. She envisioned creating personalized meal plans tailored to each patient's unique needs, taking into account their individual biochemistry and cultural preferences.

Herbal remedies, carefully selected and formulated based on their time-honored use in various healing traditions, would complement the dietary changes. From adaptogenic herbs that helped the body cope with stress to thyroid-stimulating botanicals, these natural compounds held the potential to gently nudge the body back into balance.

Mindfulness practices, such as meditation, gentle yoga, and breathwork, would be woven into the treatment plan, acknowledging the profound impact of stress and emotional turmoil on thyroid function. By cultivating inner peace and emotional resilience, patients would be better equipped to navigate the challenges of their healing journey.

As Dr. Wells gazed upon the vibrant garden, she felt a profound sense of gratitude for the wisdom of the ancients and the generosity of nature. She knew that the path ahead would be challenging, but she was determined to blaze a trail that would inspire others to embrace a holistic approach to wellness.

With a renewed sense of purpose, she turned her attention to the task at hand – refining her treatment protocols, assembling a team of like-minded practitioners, and preparing to welcome those seeking a more natural and comprehensive approach to thyroid health.

The journey had only just begun, but Dr. Wells felt a deep sense of conviction that she was on the right path – a path that would not only heal the body but also nourish the soul, fostering a harmonious balance that would empower her patients to reclaim their vitality and embrace a life of radiant well-being.

Chapter 4: Forging a New Approach

4.1 Dietary Transformations

As Dr. Wells delved deeper into her research, she discovered that diet played a crucial role in managing hypothyroidism. The conventional approach often overlooked the profound impact that food choices could have on thyroid function and overall well-being.

In her quest for natural solutions, Dr. Wells immersed herself in the study of nutritional science, exploring the intricate relationship between the foods we consume and the delicate balance of hormones within the body. She pored over ancient texts, modern research, and the wisdom of traditional healing practices, seeking to unravel the mysteries of how dietary changes could alleviate the symptoms of hypothyroidism.

One of the first revelations that struck Dr. Wells was the importance of eliminating inflammatory foods from her patients' diets. Many individuals with hypothyroidism suffered from chronic inflammation, which exacerbated their symptoms and hindered the body's ability to function optimally. By identifying and removing common inflammatory triggers such as gluten, dairy, and processed foods, she witnessed remarkable improvements in her patients' energy levels, digestion, and overall well-being.

"Food is not just fuel; it is information that speaks to our cells," Dr. Wells often reminded her patients. "By choosing the right foods, we can create an environment that supports healing and balance within our bodies."

Dr. Wells also recognized the significance of incorporating nutrient-dense, thyroid-friendly foods into her patients' diets. She encouraged the consumption of foods rich in iodine, selenium, zinc, and omega-3 fatty acids, all of which played crucial roles in supporting thyroid function. Seaweed, Brazil nuts, fatty fish, and avocados became staples in her recommended meal plans.

However, Dr. Wells understood that dietary changes alone were not a panacea. She emphasized the importance of addressing the root causes of hypothyroidism, which often involved addressing imbalances in the gut microbiome, managing stress levels, and addressing environmental toxins. By taking a holistic approach, she aimed to create a comprehensive healing strategy tailored to each individual's unique needs.

One of the most significant challenges Dr. Wells faced was helping her patients overcome deeply ingrained dietary habits and misconceptions. Many had grown accustomed to the Standard American Diet, rich in processed foods and devoid of essential nutrients. Breaking free from these patterns required patience, education, and unwavering support.

"Changing your diet is not just about the food on your plate," Dr. Wells explained. "It's about transforming your relationship with food, understanding its power to heal, and embracing a new way of nourishing your body and soul."

To facilitate this transformation, Dr. Wells developed comprehensive dietary guidelines and meal plans tailored to each patient's needs and preferences. She provided cooking classes, recipe books, and personalized consultations, empowering her patients to take control of their health through the foods they consumed.

As her patients began to incorporate these dietary changes, the results were nothing short of remarkable. Many reported increased energy levels, improved digestion, and a newfound sense of vitality. Weight management became easier, and symptoms such as brain fog, hair loss, and mood swings began to subside.

One patient, Sarah, a 35-year-old mother of two, had struggled with hypothyroidism for years. Despite being on medication, she constantly felt fatigued and struggled with her weight. After implementing Dr.

Wells's dietary recommendations, she experienced a profound transformation.

"It was like a veil had been lifted," Sarah shared. "I had no idea how much my diet was contributing to my symptoms. Now, I feel like I have my life back. I have energy to play with my kids, and I've finally been able to lose those stubborn pounds."

Dr. Wells's approach to dietary transformations was not just about treating hypothyroidism; it was about empowering her patients to reclaim their health and embrace a holistic lifestyle. By nourishing their bodies with whole, nutrient-dense foods, they were laying the foundation for lasting wellness and vitality.

As word of her success spread, more and more patients sought out Dr. Wells's guidance, eager to embark on their own journeys of dietary transformation. Each success story fueled her determination to continue pushing the boundaries of conventional medicine and spreading the message of the healing power of food.

4.2 The Power of Herbs

As Dr. Wells delved deeper into the ancient wisdom of natural healing, she discovered a treasure trove of herbal remedies that had been overlooked by modern medicine. These plant-based allies, carefully cultivated and revered by countless generations, held the potential to unlock the body's innate ability to heal and restore balance.

One of the first herbs she explored was Ashwagandha, an adaptogenic root that had been used in Ayurvedic medicine for centuries. Known for its ability to combat stress and support the endocrine system, Ashwagandha quickly became a cornerstone of her thyroid treatment protocols. Dr. Wells witnessed firsthand how this ancient herb helped her patients manage the debilitating fatigue and anxiety that often accompanied hypothyroidism.

Next, she turned her attention to the humble Bladderwrack, a nutrient-rich seaweed that had been traditionally used to support thyroid function. Rich in iodine, a mineral essential for proper thyroid hormone production, Bladderwrack provided a natural source of this vital nutrient without the potential side effects associated with synthetic supplements.

As her knowledge expanded, Dr. Wells discovered the synergistic power of combining different herbs. She crafted carefully formulated blends, each tailored to address specific symptoms and imbalances. One such blend included Rhodiola, a potent adaptogen that helped combat the brain fog and cognitive impairment that many of her patients struggled with. Combined with the calming properties of Lemon Balm and the mood-boosting effects of St. John's Wort, this herbal blend offered a comprehensive approach to supporting mental clarity and emotional well-being.

For those grappling with the weight fluctuations often associated with thyroid disorders, Dr. Wells turned to herbs like Green Tea and Garcinia Cambogia. These natural ingredients not only supported healthy metabolism but also helped curb cravings and promote a sense of fullness, making it easier for her patients to maintain a balanced diet.

Throughout her journey, Dr. Wells remained mindful of the importance of sourcing high-quality, organic herbs. She established partnerships with reputable growers and suppliers, ensuring that her patients received the purest and most potent forms of these natural remedies.

One of the most profound discoveries Dr. Wells made was the power of herbal teas. She created customized blends that not only provided therapeutic benefits but also offered a soothing ritual for her patients. The act of preparing and sipping these fragrant brews became a moment of respite, a way to connect with nature's healing energy and nurture the mind, body, and spirit.

As word of her innovative approach spread, patients from far and wide sought out Dr. Wells's expertise. She took the time to educate each individual on the properties and benefits of the herbs she prescribed, empowering them to take an active role in their healing journey.

One such patient was Emily, a young woman who had struggled with hypothyroidism since her teenage years. After years of relying on synthetic medications that left her feeling drained and disconnected,

Emily embraced Dr. Wells's herbal protocols with open arms. Within weeks of incorporating herbs like Ginseng and Schisandra into her daily routine, Emily noticed a remarkable improvement in her energy levels and overall sense of well-being.

"It's like I've been given a second chance at life," Emily shared, her eyes brimming with tears of gratitude. "For the first time in years, I feel alive again, and it's all thanks to the power of these incredible plants."

Dr. Wells's heart swelled with pride as she witnessed the transformative impact of her work. Each success story fueled her determination to continue exploring the vast realm of herbal medicine, uncovering new pathways to healing and empowering her patients to reclaim their vitality.

As the sun set over the bustling city, Dr. Wells would often find herself in her garden, surrounded by the very herbs that had become her allies in this remarkable journey. With each gentle caress of a leaf or inhale of a fragrant bloom, she felt a deep connection to the ancient wisdom that had guided her thus far. It was a reminder that nature held the answers, and it was her sacred duty to uncover and share these gifts with those who sought solace in their embrace.

4.3 The Power of Herbs

As Dr. Wells delved deeper into the ancient wisdom of natural healing, she discovered a treasure trove of herbal remedies that had been overlooked by modern medicine. These plant-based medicines, revered for centuries by various cultures, held the potential to alleviate the symptoms of hypothyroidism and restore balance to the body.

One of the first herbs she encountered was Ashwagandha, an adaptogenic herb that had been used in Ayurvedic medicine for thousands of years. Dr. Wells learned that Ashwagandha could help regulate thyroid function, reduce stress, and improve overall vitality. She began incorporating this powerful herb into her patients' treatment plans, and the results were remarkable.

"I had been struggling with fatigue and brain fog for years," recalled Sarah, one of Dr. Wells's patients. "Within weeks of taking

Ashwagandha, I felt like a fog had lifted. I had more energy, and my mind felt clearer."

Another herb that caught Dr. Wells's attention was Bladderwrack, a type of seaweed rich in iodine – a mineral essential for proper thyroid function. Many of her patients were deficient in iodine, which could exacerbate hypothyroidism symptoms. By supplementing with Bladderwrack, Dr. Wells witnessed a significant improvement in her patients' thyroid hormone levels and overall well-being.

"I had tried countless synthetic medications, but nothing seemed to work," said Mark, another patient. "When Dr. Wells introduced Bladderwrack into my treatment plan, it was like a switch had been flipped. My energy levels improved, and I finally felt like myself again."

As her knowledge of herbal medicine grew, Dr. Wells began to explore the synergistic effects of combining various herbs. She discovered that by carefully blending different plants, she could create powerful formulations that targeted multiple aspects of hypothyroidism.

One such formulation included Guggul, an Ayurvedic herb known for its ability to support thyroid function, along with Selenium, a mineral that played a crucial role in the production of thyroid hormones. This combination proved to be a game-changer for many of her patients, helping to regulate their thyroid levels and alleviate symptoms such as weight gain and hair loss.

"I had tried every diet and exercise regimen imaginable, but nothing seemed to help me lose weight," recalled Emily, a long-time patient. "Within a few months of taking Dr. Wells's herbal formulation, the pounds started melting away. It was like a miracle."

In addition to these powerful herbs, Dr. Wells also incorporated adaptogens like Rhodiola and Ginseng into her treatment plans. These herbs helped her patients cope with the stress and fatigue that often accompanied hypothyroidism, promoting a sense of balance and well-being.

As word of Dr. Wells's innovative approach spread, more and more patients sought her out, eager to explore the healing power of nature.

She took the time to educate each individual on the benefits and proper use of the herbs, ensuring that they understood the importance of a holistic approach to their health.

"Dr. Wells didn't just hand me a bottle of pills and send me on my way," said Jessica, a grateful patient. "She took the time to explain how each herb worked and how it would complement the other aspects of my treatment plan. I felt empowered and in control of my own healing journey."

With each passing day, Dr. Wells witnessed the transformative effects of herbal medicine on her patients' lives. Their renewed energy, improved mood, and overall vitality were a testament to the power of nature's bounty.

However, she knew that her work was far from over. The medical establishment remained skeptical of her unconventional approach, and she would need to continue advocating for the integration of natural remedies into mainstream healthcare.

But for now, Dr. Wells found solace in the grateful smiles and heartfelt testimonies of her patients. She had rediscovered the ancient wisdom of herbal healing, and with it, she had unlocked a path to wellness that had been forgotten by modern medicine.

As she looked to the future, Dr. Wells felt a renewed sense of purpose. She would continue to champion the power of herbs, spreading their healing magic to those in need, and paving the way for a more holistic approach to healthcare.

4.4 Harnessing Inner Strength

As Dr. Wells delved deeper into the realm of holistic healing, she realized that the mind and body were inextricably linked. The physical symptoms of hypothyroidism were often exacerbated by emotional and psychological factors, creating a vicious cycle that could be challenging to break. To truly address the root causes of thyroid disorders, she knew she had to incorporate practices that nurtured the mind and spirit.

One of the first techniques Dr. Wells introduced to her patients was mindfulness meditation. She had long been fascinated by the ancient practice of cultivating present-moment awareness, and she believed it could be a powerful tool in managing the stress and anxiety that often accompanied thyroid conditions.

Initially, some patients were skeptical about the benefits of meditation. They had come seeking tangible solutions, not esoteric practices. However, Dr. Wells gently encouraged them to approach it with an open mind, explaining that reducing stress levels could have a profound impact on their overall well-being.

During the guided meditation sessions, Dr. Wells led her patients through a series of breathing exercises and visualization techniques. She encouraged them to focus on the present moment, letting go of worries about the past or future. As they practiced this mindful awareness, many patients reported feeling a sense of calm wash over them, a respite from the constant chatter of their minds.

"At first, I found it challenging to quiet my thoughts," confessed Samantha, a patient who had been struggling with hypothyroidism for years. "But as I continued practicing, I noticed that I could approach each day with a greater sense of clarity and resilience."

In addition to mindfulness meditation, Dr. Wells incorporated other stress-reduction techniques into her treatment plans. She introduced gentle yoga practices, emphasizing the importance of connecting with one's breath and cultivating a sense of self-awareness. The soothing movements and deep breathing exercises helped patients release physical tension while promoting a state of relaxation.

For those who found it difficult to quiet their minds during traditional meditation, Dr. Wells suggested journaling as an alternative outlet. Writing down thoughts and emotions could be a cathartic experience, allowing patients to process their feelings and gain insight into the underlying emotional patterns that might be contributing to their condition.

As her patients embraced these mind-body practices, Dr. Wells witnessed remarkable transformations. Patients who had previously felt overwhelmed by their symptoms began to develop a newfound sense of resilience and inner strength. They reported improved sleep quality, reduced anxiety, and a greater ability to manage stress – all of which had a positive impact on their overall health and well-being.

"It's not just about treating the physical symptoms," Dr. Wells explained. "True healing requires addressing the whole person – mind, body, and spirit. By cultivating inner strength and resilience, we can better navigate the challenges that come with thyroid disorders and reclaim our vitality."

One patient, Emily, had been struggling with hypothyroidism for years, and the constant fatigue and brain fog had taken a toll on her mental health. After incorporating mindfulness practices into her treatment plan, she experienced a profound shift.

"For the first time in years, I feel like I'm in control of my life again," Emily shared, her eyes shining with newfound hope. "The meditation and journaling have helped me process the emotions I've been carrying, and I've gained a deeper understanding of myself. I'm no longer just surviving – I'm truly living."

As word of Dr. Wells's holistic approach spread, more and more patients sought her guidance, eager to explore the power of mind-body practices in their healing journeys. While the path was not always easy, the transformations they witnessed in themselves and others served as a testament to the profound impact of harnessing inner strength.

Dr. Wells knew that this was just the beginning. By integrating these ancient wisdom traditions with modern medical knowledge, she was paving the way for a new era of healthcare – one that recognized the interconnectedness of mind, body, and spirit, and empowered individuals to take an active role in their own healing process.

4.5 Integrating the Pieces

As Dr. Wells delved deeper into the realm of natural healing, she realized that true wellness could not be achieved through a single modality alone.

It required a harmonious integration of various holistic approaches, each complementing the other in a symphony of healing.

The key to her pioneering approach was the recognition that every individual was unique, with distinct needs and imbalances. A one-size-fits-all solution was not only ineffective but also counterproductive. Instead, Dr. Wells crafted personalized treatment plans that addressed the root causes of hypothyroidism while nurturing the body's innate ability to heal itself.

The first step in this integrative process was to understand the patient's unique biochemistry and lifestyle. Through comprehensive assessments and open conversations, Dr. Wells sought to unravel the intricate web of factors contributing to their condition. From dietary habits and environmental exposures to emotional stressors and genetic predispositions, no stone was left unturned.

With this holistic understanding, Dr. Wells began to weave together a tapestry of natural therapies tailored to each individual's needs. Dietary modifications played a pivotal role, as she guided her patients towards nutrient-dense, anti-inflammatory foods that supported thyroid function and overall well-being. Herbal supplements were carefully selected, harnessing the power of nature's bounty to gently restore balance and vitality.

Acupuncture, an ancient healing art rooted in the principles of energy flow, became an integral part of her approach. By stimulating specific points along the body's meridians, Dr. Wells helped to remove blockages and restore the harmonious flow of vital energy, promoting optimal thyroid function and overall health.

However, Dr. Wells understood that physical healing was only one aspect of the journey. She recognized the profound impact of stress and emotional turmoil on the body's delicate balance. To address this, she incorporated mindfulness practices, such as meditation and breathwork, into her treatment plans. These techniques not only helped her patients manage stress but also cultivated a deeper connection with their inner selves, fostering self-awareness and emotional resilience.

As her patients embraced this multifaceted approach, they began to experience profound transformations. The integration of these various modalities created a synergistic effect, amplifying the healing potential of each individual component. Fatigue gave way to renewed vitality, emotional turmoil transformed into inner peace, and physical ailments gradually subsided.

Dr. Wells's integrative approach was not merely a collection of disparate therapies but rather a harmonious symphony, where each element played a vital role in restoring balance and promoting holistic well-being. It was a testament to the power of nature's wisdom and the body's innate capacity to heal when given the right support and guidance.

Through her pioneering work, Dr. Wells challenged the conventional paradigm of treating hypothyroidism with synthetic medications alone. She demonstrated that true healing could be achieved by embracing a holistic approach that addressed the root causes of imbalance and nurtured the body's innate wisdom.

As word of her remarkable success spread, more and more individuals sought out Dr. Wells's integrative care, eager to embark on their own journeys of healing and transformation. Her clinic became a beacon of hope, a sanctuary where the ancient wisdom of natural healing intertwined with modern scientific understanding, offering a path towards lasting wellness and vitality.

Chapter 5: Healing Journeys

5.1 Renewed Vitality

As the first rays of sunlight filtered through the curtains, Emily stirred in her bed, her eyes fluttering open. For the first time in years, she felt a sense of lightness and energy coursing through her body. The fog that had once enveloped her mind had lifted, and she greeted the day with a newfound clarity.

Emily had been one of Dr. Wells's earliest patients, a woman in her thirties who had been struggling with hypothyroidism for over a decade. She had tried countless medications and treatments, but nothing seemed to alleviate the overwhelming fatigue and brain fog that had become her constant companions.

When she first stepped into Dr. Wells's clinic, Emily was skeptical. She had heard about the naturopath's unconventional approach and was hesitant to embrace yet another treatment that promised relief but might fail to deliver. However, as she listened to Dr. Wells's compassionate explanations and holistic philosophy, a glimmer of hope began to kindle within her.

The first step in Emily's journey was a complete overhaul of her diet. Dr. Wells emphasized the importance of eliminating inflammatory foods and incorporating nutrient-dense, thyroid-friendly options. Emily bid farewell to processed foods, gluten, and dairy, and embraced a vibrant array of fresh fruits, vegetables, and lean proteins.

Initially, the dietary changes were challenging, but Emily's determination to reclaim her vitality propelled her forward. She meticulously planned her meals, experimenting with new recipes and flavors that nourished her body and soul.

Alongside the dietary changes, Dr. Wells introduced Emily to a carefully curated blend of herbal supplements. These natural remedies, derived from ancient wisdom and modern research, were designed to support and nourish her thyroid function.

Emily diligently followed the recommended dosages, and within a few weeks, she began to notice subtle shifts in her energy levels. The constant fatigue that had once weighed her down started to dissipate, and she found herself able to stay focused and alert throughout the day.

As the weeks turned into months, Emily's transformation became increasingly apparent. Her once-dull complexion regained a healthy glow, and the brain fog that had plagued her for years slowly lifted, allowing her to think clearly and sharply.

Encouraged by her progress, Emily embraced the other aspects of Dr. Wells's holistic approach. She began practicing gentle yoga and meditation, techniques that helped her manage stress and cultivate a sense of inner peace. The acupuncture sessions, initially daunting, became a source of profound relaxation and balance.

With each passing day, Emily felt herself becoming stronger, more vibrant, and more alive. The debilitating fatigue that had once defined her existence was now a distant memory, replaced by a newfound zest for life.

During her follow-up appointments, Dr. Wells beamed with pride as she witnessed Emily's remarkable transformation. The woman who had once walked through the clinic's doors with a weary gait and sunken eyes now radiated energy and vitality.

Emily's story became a beacon of hope for other patients struggling with hypothyroidism. Her journey inspired them to embrace the holistic approach wholeheartedly, trusting in the power of nature and the body's innate ability to heal when given the proper support.

As Emily shared her experiences with others, she became an advocate for Dr. Wells's integrative methods. Her testimony resonated deeply with those who had endured similar struggles, offering them a glimmer of hope that they, too, could reclaim their vitality and live life to the fullest.

In the bustling clinic, Emily's radiant smile and infectious energy became a symbol of the transformative power of holistic healing. Her journey was a testament to the efficacy of Dr. Wells's approach and a reminder that even the most daunting challenges could be overcome with perseverance, knowledge, and a deep respect for the wisdom of nature.

5.2 Shedding the Weight

For years, Sarah had watched her patients struggle with the frustrating battle against weight gain, a common symptom of hypothyroidism. Despite their best efforts, the numbers on the scale seemed to creep up relentlessly, leaving them feeling defeated and discouraged.

One such patient was Emily, a vibrant young woman whose zest for life had been dimmed by the constant struggle with her weight. At their initial consultation, Emily's eyes were filled with tears as she recounted her journey.

"I've tried every diet under the sun," she confessed. "I've counted calories, cut out carbs, and even tried extreme fasting, but nothing seems to work. It's like my body is fighting against me."

Sarah listened intently, recognizing the all-too-familiar story. She knew that conventional weight loss approaches often fell short for those with thyroid imbalances, as the root cause remained unaddressed.

With a gentle smile, Sarah reassured Emily, "I understand how disheartening this must feel, but there is hope. Together, we'll explore a holistic approach that addresses the underlying issue and supports your body's natural ability to achieve a healthy weight."

The first step in Emily's journey was to adopt a thyroid-friendly diet. Sarah emphasized the importance of nutrient-dense, anti-inflammatory foods that could support optimal thyroid function. She introduced Emily to the concept of eliminating foods that could potentially exacerbate inflammation and disrupt hormone balance.

Initially, the dietary changes seemed daunting to Emily, but Sarah's guidance and encouragement made the transition smoother. Slowly but surely, Emily began to incorporate more whole, unprocessed foods into her meals, favoring options like leafy greens, fatty fish, and fermented foods.

Alongside the dietary adjustments, Sarah recommended a carefully selected blend of herbal supplements to support Emily's thyroid health. These natural remedies, derived from ancient wisdom and modern research, aimed to gently nudge her body back into balance.

As the weeks passed, Emily noticed a gradual shift. The brain fog that had plagued her began to lift, and her energy levels started to improve. But perhaps the most remarkable change was the way her body responded to the holistic approach.

"It's like a weight has been lifted, both literally and figuratively," Emily exclaimed during one of her follow-up appointments. "The numbers on the scale are finally moving in the right direction, and I feel like I'm regaining control over my health."

Sarah beamed with pride, witnessing the transformation unfold before her eyes. Emily's success was a testament to the power of nature's thyroid solution, a gentle yet effective approach that addressed the root cause rather than merely treating the symptoms.

For others like Emily, the journey to shedding excess weight was often a winding path, with its share of challenges and setbacks. But Sarah remained steadfast in her belief that a holistic, personalized approach could make all the difference.

Take the case of Mark, a middle-aged businessman whose demanding career had taken a toll on his health. Years of stress, poor dietary choices, and a sedentary lifestyle had contributed to his weight gain and exacerbated his hypothyroidism.

When Mark first stepped into Sarah's clinic, he was skeptical about the idea of natural remedies. "I've tried every pill and potion out there," he remarked, his voice tinged with resignation. "Nothing seems to work for me."

Sarah understood his skepticism but remained undeterred. She carefully crafted a comprehensive plan for Mark, addressing not only his dietary needs but also incorporating stress-reduction techniques and gentle exercise routines.

"Healing is a journey, and it requires patience and commitment," Sarah explained. "But with the right tools and support, your body has an incredible ability to heal itself."

Slowly but surely, Mark began to embrace the holistic approach. He traded his fast-food lunches for nutrient-dense salads and incorporated mindfulness practices into his daily routine. As the weeks turned into months, the changes became evident – not only in his weight but also in his overall well-being.

"I never thought I'd say this, but I actually look forward to my morning walks," Mark confessed during one of his follow-up visits. "It's like a fog has lifted, and I can finally see the path to a healthier, happier me."

Sarah's heart swelled with joy as she witnessed the transformations unfolding before her. Each success story reinforced her belief in the power of nature's thyroid solution and the importance of addressing the root cause of imbalance.

As she looked around her clinic, filled with patients embarking on their own healing journeys, Sarah knew that her mission was far from over. There were countless others out there, struggling with the weight of hypothyroidism, waiting to be guided towards a holistic path to wellness.

With renewed determination, Sarah vowed to continue spreading the message of natural healing, one patient at a time, until the world embraced the transformative power of nature's thyroid solution.

5.3 Emotional Equilibrium

For years, Sarah had witnessed the profound impact hypothyroidism had on her patients' emotional well-being. The hormonal imbalances caused by the condition often manifested as mood swings, anxiety, and even depression. Conventional treatments, while addressing the physical symptoms, fell short in restoring the delicate emotional equilibrium her patients so desperately sought.

It was during her exploration of ancient healing traditions that Sarah stumbled upon a remarkable discovery – the intricate connection between the thyroid gland and the body's emotional center. In the ancient texts, she found references to the thyroid as the "gland of emotion," a vital regulator of mood and mental clarity.

Inspired by these insights, Sarah began incorporating holistic practices into her treatment plans, aimed at nurturing not just the physical but also the emotional and spiritual aspects of her patients' well-being.

One such practice was the ancient art of meditation. Sarah introduced her patients to various meditation techniques, tailored to their individual needs and preferences. For some, it was the calming practice of mindfulness meditation, allowing them to anchor their thoughts in the present moment and find solace amidst the chaos of their minds. For others, it was the gentle guidance of guided imagery, where they could visualize themselves in a state of tranquility and inner peace.

Sarah witnessed the transformative power of meditation firsthand. Patients who had once struggled with overwhelming anxiety and mood swings gradually found a sense of calm and emotional balance. The simple act of quieting the mind and focusing on the breath proved to be a potent tool in managing the emotional turmoil that often accompanied hypothyroidism.

Alongside meditation, Sarah introduced her patients to the healing benefits of aromatherapy. She carefully selected essential oils known for their calming and uplifting properties, such as lavender, bergamot, and ylang-ylang. These fragrant allies were incorporated into massage oils, diffusers, and even bath salts, creating a multi-sensory experience that soothed the mind and nourished the soul.

As her patients embraced these holistic practices, Sarah noticed a remarkable shift in their demeanor. The once-weary expressions were replaced by radiant smiles, and the heavy burdens they carried seemed to lighten with each passing day.

One such patient was Emily, a young mother who had struggled with postpartum depression and anxiety for months after the birth of her second child. Despite being on medication, Emily felt disconnected from her own emotions, unable to fully embrace the joys of motherhood.

Sarah introduced Emily to a combination of meditation, aromatherapy, and gentle yoga practices. At first, Emily was skeptical, but as she persisted, she began to notice subtle changes. The weight of her emotions gradually lifted, and she found herself more present and attuned to the needs of her children.

"It was like a veil had been lifted," Emily shared during one of her follow-up appointments. "For the first time in months, I felt like myself again – calm, centered, and able to fully appreciate the beauty of my life."

Sarah's heart swelled with pride as she witnessed Emily's transformation. It was a testament to the power of holistic healing and the profound impact it could have on restoring emotional balance.

As word of her innovative approach spread, more and more patients sought out Sarah's guidance, each with their own unique emotional struggles. Some grappled with the overwhelming fatigue and brain fog that often accompanied hypothyroidism, while others battled with feelings of isolation and low self-esteem.

Sarah welcomed them all with open arms, tailoring her treatment plans to address their specific needs. She combined meditation and aromatherapy with other holistic practices, such as journaling, art therapy, and support group sessions, creating a comprehensive approach to emotional healing.

Through her work, Sarah came to understand that emotional well-being was not just a byproduct of physical health but an integral part of the healing process. By addressing the emotional turmoil that often accompanied hypothyroidism, she empowered her patients to reclaim their lives and embrace a newfound sense of balance and inner peace.

As the sun set on another day at her clinic, Sarah reflected on the countless lives she had touched through her holistic approach. Each patient's journey was a testament to the power of nature, the resilience of the human spirit, and the transformative potential of embracing emotional equilibrium.

5.4 Restoring Radiance

Sarah's heart swelled with joy as she witnessed the transformative power of her holistic approach unfold before her eyes. One of her most remarkable cases was that of Amelia, a young woman whose battle with hypothyroidism had taken a toll on her once-vibrant appearance.

Amelia had been a radiant beauty, her golden locks shimmering in the sunlight and her hazel eyes sparkling with life. However, the insidious effects of hypothyroidism had slowly robbed her of her natural glow. Her hair had become dull and brittle, her complexion sallow and lifeless, and dark circles had taken up permanent residence beneath her eyes.

Despite her best efforts to conceal the outward signs of her condition, Amelia's confidence had been shattered. She felt like a mere shadow of her former self, and the once-simple act of looking in the mirror had become a source of anguish.

When Amelia first stepped into Sarah's clinic, she was a broken woman, her spirit crushed by the relentless onslaught of her symptoms. But Sarah saw beyond the physical manifestations of her condition, recognizing the radiant beauty that still resided within.

With a gentle touch and a compassionate heart, Sarah crafted a personalized treatment plan that addressed not only the physiological aspects of Amelia's condition but also the emotional and spiritual dimensions.

The first step was to overhaul Amelia's diet, eliminating inflammatory foods and incorporating nutrient-dense, thyroid-friendly options. Sarah introduced her to the healing power of herbs, carefully selecting a blend of adaptogenic and hormone-balancing botanicals to support her endocrine system.

Acupuncture sessions were woven into the treatment plan, helping to restore the flow of vital energy and alleviate the stress that had been exacerbating Amelia's symptoms. Sarah also guided her through mindfulness practices, teaching her techniques to cultivate inner peace and self-acceptance.

Week by week, Amelia's transformation unfolded like a delicate flower blooming in the spring. Her hair regained its lustrous shine, her complexion took on a healthy glow, and the dark circles beneath her eyes faded, revealing the warmth and vibrancy that had been hidden for so long.

But the true transformation extended far beyond the physical realm. Amelia's spirit was reawakened, her confidence restored, and her zest for life reignited. She began to see herself through new eyes, appreciating the unique beauty that radiated from within.

Sarah marveled at Amelia's progress, her heart swelling with pride and gratitude for the healing power of nature. Each time Amelia walked through the clinic doors, her radiant smile was a testament to the profound impact of holistic wellness.

As word of Amelia's transformation spread, others sought out Sarah's guidance, their eyes filled with hope and a yearning for the same radiant vitality. Sarah welcomed them with open arms, her passion for her work burning brighter than ever before.

In the quiet moments, Sarah would reflect on the journey that had led her to this point. She remembered the seed of doubt that had been planted in her heart, the voices of those suffering in silence, and the ancient wisdom that had guided her towards a new path.

Now, as she witnessed the transformations unfolding before her, Sarah knew that she had found her true calling. She was not merely a healer of physical ailments; she was a catalyst for profound, holistic change – a guide on a journey towards radiant wellness.

Each patient who walked through her doors was a reminder of the power of perseverance and the resilience of the human spirit. Their stories woven together into a tapestry of hope, resilience, and the indomitable strength of the human spirit.

As Amelia's laughter echoed through the clinic, Sarah felt a deep sense of fulfillment. She knew that her work was far from over, but in that moment, she was filled with gratitude for the opportunity to be a part of such profound transformations, to witness the restoration of radiance in all its glory.

5.5 Embracing Wholeness

As the weeks and months passed, Dr. Wells witnessed remarkable transformations in her patients. What had once seemed like an uphill battle against the relentless symptoms of hypothyroidism was now a testament to the power of holistic healing. Each individual's journey was unique, yet they shared a common thread – a newfound sense of wholeness that permeated every aspect of their lives.

One such patient was Emily, a young mother who had struggled with hypothyroidism since the birth of her second child. Despite following her doctor's prescribed medication regimen, she found herself trapped in a cycle of fatigue, brain fog, and emotional turmoil. The once vibrant and energetic woman she had been seemed like a distant memory.

"I felt like a shell of my former self," Emily confided in Dr. Wells during one of their sessions. "The medications helped a little, but I was still so tired all the time. I couldn't focus, and my mood swings were taking a toll on my family."

Dr. Wells listened intently, her heart aching for the suffering Emily had endured. She knew that true healing required more than just a pill – it demanded a holistic approach that addressed the root causes of Emily's condition.

Together, they embarked on a transformative journey. Dr. Wells guided Emily through dietary changes, introducing nutrient-dense foods that nourished her body and supported her thyroid function. They explored the power of adaptogenic herbs, which helped to regulate Emily's stress response and alleviate the emotional upheaval she had been experiencing.

Slowly but surely, Emily began to notice a shift. The fog that had clouded her mind started to dissipate, and her energy levels gradually increased. With the support of Dr. Wells and the holistic treatment plan, Emily rediscovered her zest for life.

"It was like waking up from a long, dark slumber," Emily shared, her eyes sparkling with newfound vitality. "I felt alive again, present in every moment with my family. The constant fatigue and mood swings were no longer holding me back."

But Emily's transformation went beyond the physical. Through her journey with Dr. Wells, she had developed a deeper appreciation for the interconnectedness of mind, body, and spirit. She had learned to listen to her body's cues, to nourish herself with wholesome foods, and to find solace in practices like meditation and gentle exercise.

"I used to think that taking a pill was the only solution," Emily admitted. "But now I understand that true healing requires a holistic approach. It's about nourishing every aspect of my being – physical, emotional, and spiritual."

Emily's story was just one of many that Dr. Wells had the privilege of witnessing. Each patient's journey was unique, but they all shared a common thread – a newfound sense of wholeness that permeated every aspect of their lives.

There was Sarah, a busy executive who had struggled with weight gain and brain fog, now reveling in her newfound energy and mental clarity. And then there was Michael, a retired teacher who had battled depression and hair loss, now embracing a renewed sense of purpose and self-confidence.

As Dr. Wells looked around her clinic, she saw a community of individuals who had once been burdened by the debilitating effects of hypothyroidism, now thriving and embracing a holistic approach to wellness. Their journeys were a testament to the power of integrative care, a harmonious blend of modern medicine and ancient wisdom.

In their eyes, Dr. Wells saw a spark of hope, a recognition that true healing was possible when the body, mind, and spirit were nurtured in equal measure. It was a profound realization that transcended the boundaries of conventional medicine, reminding her that sometimes the most profound solutions lie in the simplicity of nature's embrace.

With each success story, Dr. Wells felt a sense of deep gratitude for the path she had chosen. Her unwavering belief in the healing power of nature had not only transformed the lives of her patients but had also ignited a flame within herself – a flame that burned brighter with every triumph, fueling her determination to continue pushing the boundaries of integrative care.

As she looked towards the future, Dr. Wells knew that her work was far from over. There were countless others out there, struggling with the same challenges her patients had faced, yearning for a holistic approach that could restore their vitality and sense of wholeness.

But with each patient who embraced the transformative power of nature's thyroid solution, Dr. Wells felt a renewed sense of purpose. She was paving the way for a paradigm shift, a revolution in healthcare that celebrated the harmonious union of modern medicine and ancient wisdom. And as she gazed upon the faces of those she had helped, she knew that this was just the beginning – a spark that would ignite a fire of change, illuminating the path towards a more holistic, compassionate, and integrated approach to wellness.

Chapter 6: The Resistance Rises

6.1 Skepticism Unveiled

As Dr. Sarah Wells' holistic approach to treating hypothyroidism gained traction, she found herself facing a formidable challenge – the skepticism of the conventional medical community. The very foundation upon which she had built her practice was being called into question, and the resistance she encountered was both relentless and unyielding.

The first rumblings of doubt emerged from her colleagues within the medical establishment. Whispers of "unproven methods" and "pseudoscience" echoed through the hallways of hospitals and clinics. Dr. Wells' peers, many of whom had been trained in the traditional, pharmaceutical-driven model of healthcare, viewed her integrative approach with a mixture of curiosity and suspicion.

"How can you claim to treat a condition as complex as hypothyroidism with mere herbs and lifestyle changes?" one doctor challenged her during a heated discussion at a medical conference. "Where are the double-blind, placebo-controlled studies to support your claims?"

Dr. Wells understood their skepticism. After all, she had once been entrenched in the same mindset, relying solely on synthetic medications and conventional treatments. However, her personal journey and the transformative results she had witnessed in her patients had opened her eyes to a world of possibilities beyond the confines of mainstream medicine.

"I understand your concerns," she would respond calmly. "But I implore you to keep an open mind. The human body is a remarkable system, and nature has provided us with an abundance of healing resources that we have yet to fully explore."

Despite her attempts to engage in respectful dialogue, the resistance only seemed to intensify. Certain medical associations began to scrutinize her practice, questioning the legality of her methods and the validity of her credentials. Accusations of practicing medicine without a license and making unsubstantiated claims were leveled against her, casting a shadow of doubt over her life's work.

Yet, Dr. Wells remained steadfast in her convictions. She knew that the true skeptics were those who refused to acknowledge the limitations of the conventional approach and the potential of alternative therapies. With each challenge, she became more determined to prove the efficacy of her methods and to advocate for a more holistic understanding of health and wellness.

"We cannot continue to treat the human body as a mere collection of parts, addressing symptoms with synthetic compounds while ignoring the root causes," she would assert. "True healing requires a comprehensive approach that addresses the mind, body, and spirit as a interconnected whole."

As the controversy swirled around her, Dr. Wells found solace in the testimonies of her patients. Their stories of transformation, from debilitating fatigue to renewed vitality, from emotional turmoil to inner peace, served as a powerful validation of her work. These individuals, once dismissed by the conventional medical system as hopeless cases, had found healing through the very methods that were now being questioned.

"Dr. Wells saved my life," one patient declared, her eyes shining with gratitude. "After years of suffering from hypothyroidism and its countless symptoms, I finally found relief through her holistic approach. I am living proof that nature has the power to heal, if we only have the courage to embrace it."

Such testimonies fueled Dr. Wells' determination to persevere in the face of skepticism. She knew that the path she had chosen was not an easy one, but it was a necessary journey – a quest to challenge the status quo and pave the way for a more inclusive, integrative approach to healthcare.

As the resistance mounted, Dr. Wells found herself at a crossroads. She could either retreat into the shadows, abandoning her principles and conforming to the expectations of the medical establishment, or she could stand firm, weathering the storm and continuing to advocate for a paradigm shift in the way we perceive and treat thyroid disorders.

With unwavering resolve, she chose the latter path, ready to confront the skepticism head-on and prove that nature's thyroid solution was not only viable but essential in the pursuit of true healing.

6.2 Defending the Unconventional

As Dr. Wells's integrative approach to treating hypothyroidism gained traction, she found herself facing an increasingly vocal opposition from the conventional medical establishment. The skepticism she encountered was not entirely unexpected, but the intensity and persistence of the resistance caught her off guard.

The first wave of criticism came from her former colleagues at the prestigious Metropolis Medical Center, where she had once been a respected physician. Whispers of "quackery" and "pseudoscience" echoed through the hallways, and some even questioned her medical credentials.

"Sarah, you were once a brilliant doctor," Dr. Evan Sinclair, her former mentor, admonished during a heated exchange. "How can you abandon evidence-based medicine for these unproven, alternative therapies?"

Dr. Wells remained steadfast in her convictions. "Evan, I understand your concerns, but the evidence is right in front of us. My patients are experiencing remarkable improvements using these natural approaches. Isn't that what truly matters?"

Sinclair shook his head, his brow furrowed with skepticism. "Anecdotal evidence is not enough. You need to conduct proper clinical trials and submit your findings for peer review."

Dr. Wells knew he had a point. While she had meticulously documented her patients' progress, she lacked the resources and funding to conduct large-scale studies. Nevertheless, she refused to dismiss the transformative results she had witnessed firsthand.

The criticism extended beyond her former colleagues. Local medical associations and regulatory bodies began scrutinizing her practice, questioning the legality of her unconventional treatments. Letters demanding explanations and justifications piled up on her desk, each one more ominous than the last.

Despite the mounting pressure, Dr. Wells remained resolute. She understood that challenging the status quo often came at a price, but she was unwilling to compromise her principles or abandon her patients.

"I will not back down," she declared to her staff during a tense meeting. "We are on the cusp of a paradigm shift in healthcare, and we must stand firm in our beliefs."

Her unwavering determination inspired her team, and they rallied behind her, united in their commitment to holistic healing. Together, they began compiling research, gathering evidence from reputable sources, and meticulously documenting their patients' progress.

Dr. Wells also sought support from like-minded professionals around the world. She attended conferences, participated in webinars, and engaged in lively discussions with pioneers in the field of integrative medicine. Through these connections, she gained invaluable insights and fortified her resolve.

One such ally was Dr. Amara Patel, a renowned naturopathic physician from India. During a video conference, Dr. Patel shared her own experiences battling skepticism and resistance.

"The path you have chosen is not an easy one, my friend," she said, her voice carrying the weight of hard-earned wisdom. "But remember, true progress often comes at the cost of discomfort. Embrace the resistance, for it is a testament to the impact you are making."

Emboldened by Dr. Patel's words, Dr. Wells redoubled her efforts to defend her unconventional approach. She organized public seminars, wrote articles for medical journals, and even appeared on local television programs, passionately advocating for the integration of natural remedies into mainstream healthcare.

As the debate intensified, Dr. Wells found herself at the center of a growing movement. Patients who had experienced the transformative power of her treatments became vocal advocates, sharing their stories and lending their voices to the cause.

One such patient was Emily Thompson, a young woman who had struggled with hypothyroidism for years before finding relief through Dr. Wells's holistic approach.

"Dr. Wells gave me back my life," Emily proclaimed during a public forum. "After years of taking synthetic medications with minimal results, her natural remedies finally allowed me to reclaim my energy, lose the excess weight, and regain my zest for living."

Stories like Emily's resonated with the public, and support for Dr. Wells's work began to swell. While the medical establishment remained skeptical, a growing number of individuals embraced the idea of integrating natural therapies into their healthcare regimens.

Through it all, Dr. Wells remained steadfast in her belief that true healing required a holistic approach, one that addressed the root causes of illness rather than merely treating symptoms. She was determined to defend the unconventional, not for personal gain, but for the sake of her patients and the countless others who sought a more natural path to wellness.

6.3 Navigating the System

As Dr. Wells's holistic approach to treating hypothyroidism gained traction, she found herself navigating a complex and often rigid medical system. The conventional healthcare establishment, rooted in its long-standing traditions and protocols, viewed her unconventional methods with skepticism and resistance.

The first hurdle she encountered was the lack of recognition for naturopathic medicine within the mainstream healthcare system. Despite her extensive training and expertise, Dr. Wells's credentials were often questioned or dismissed by her colleagues in conventional medicine. She found herself having to justify her qualifications time and time again, even as her patients experienced remarkable improvements under her care.

"It's disheartening to have your knowledge and experience constantly scrutinized," Dr. Wells confided to a colleague. "We're all striving for the same goal – to help our patients heal. Why can't we embrace different approaches that yield positive results?"

Undeterred, Dr. Wells sought to bridge the gap between her holistic practices and the conventional medical system. She understood that true progress could only be achieved through collaboration and open-mindedness on both sides.

One of her first steps was to establish a network of like-minded healthcare professionals who shared her vision for integrative medicine. This network provided a supportive community where they could exchange ideas, share research, and collectively advocate for the recognition of alternative therapies.

"We can't operate in silos," Dr. Wells emphasized during one of their meetings. "By joining forces, we amplify our voices and increase our chances of effecting real change within the system."

However, navigating the bureaucratic maze of the healthcare industry proved to be a formidable challenge. Dr. Wells found herself grappling with a myriad of regulations, insurance policies, and administrative hurdles that often hindered her ability to provide the care her patients deserved.

Insurance companies, bound by strict guidelines and protocols, were reluctant to cover many of the natural remedies and alternative therapies she prescribed. This meant that her patients had to bear the financial burden of seeking holistic treatment, which was not always feasible for those with limited resources.

"It's a vicious cycle," Dr. Wells lamented. "The system is designed to favor conventional medicine, making it difficult for patients to access alternative treatments, even when those treatments have proven effective."

Undaunted, Dr. Wells navigated these obstacles with a combination of perseverance and strategic thinking. She worked tirelessly to educate insurance providers about the benefits and cost-effectiveness of her approach, presenting them with research and case studies that demonstrated the long-term savings and improved quality of life for her patients.

She also sought to collaborate with conventional medical practitioners, inviting them to observe her clinic's operations and witness firsthand the positive impact of her integrative approach. While some remained skeptical, others were intrigued by the promising results and open to exploring new avenues of treatment.

"We can't dismiss something simply because it challenges our preconceived notions," remarked Dr. Jenkins, a respected endocrinologist who had initially been skeptical of Dr. Wells's methods. "If it works and improves the lives of our patients, we owe it to them to keep an open mind."

As Dr. Wells continued to navigate the complexities of the healthcare system, she remained steadfast in her commitment to providing her patients with the best possible care. She understood that true change often came slowly, but she was willing to persevere, one patient and one open-minded healthcare professional at a time.

"Change is never easy," she reflected. "But when we have the courage to challenge the status quo and embrace new perspectives, we open the door to transformative possibilities – for our patients, for our profession, and for the future of healthcare."

With her unwavering determination and a growing network of supporters, Dr. Wells was paving the way for a more inclusive and integrative approach to healthcare, one that recognized the value of both conventional and alternative therapies in the pursuit of holistic wellness.

6.4 Staying True to Principles

As the whispers of skepticism grew louder, Dr. Wells found herself at a crossroads. The conventional medical establishment, with its deeply entrenched beliefs and protocols, viewed her holistic approach as a threat to the status quo. Yet, she remained unwavering in her conviction that nature held the key to healing thyroid disorders.

The first wave of criticism came from within her own profession. Colleagues who had once been supportive now expressed doubts about her methods, citing a lack of empirical evidence and clinical trials. They questioned the efficacy of herbal remedies and dismissed the ancient wisdom she had uncovered as mere folklore.

"Sarah, we understand your desire to explore alternative treatments," one colleague remarked during a heated discussion. "But you must recognize that modern medicine is built upon rigorous scientific research. Without controlled studies and peer-reviewed data, how can we trust these unconventional methods?"

Dr. Wells listened patiently, her resolve unshaken. She understood the importance of scientific validation, but she also recognized the limitations of a system that often overlooked the holistic nature of healing.

"I respect the principles of evidence-based medicine," she replied calmly. "However, we must also acknowledge that our current understanding of the human body and its intricate workings is far from complete. Nature has provided us with a vast array of remedies, many of which have been used for centuries by various cultures. To dismiss them outright would be a disservice to the pursuit of knowledge."

As the debates raged on, Dr. Wells found solace in the testimonies of her patients. Their remarkable transformations, achieved through a combination of natural therapies and lifestyle changes, were undeniable. The renewed vitality in their eyes, the lightness in their steps, and the genuine smiles that graced their faces were the most compelling evidence she could offer.

"Dr. Wells, I cannot thank you enough," one patient confided, tears of gratitude glistening in her eyes. "For years, I struggled with the debilitating effects of hypothyroidism, feeling like a mere shadow of my former self. Your holistic approach has not only alleviated my physical symptoms but has also restored my emotional well-being. I feel alive again."

Such heartfelt expressions of gratitude fueled Dr. Wells's determination to stay the course. She understood that her principles were not merely a matter of personal belief but a testament to the power of nature and the inherent wisdom of the human body.

As the scrutiny intensified, Dr. Wells found herself navigating a complex web of regulations and bureaucratic hurdles. Certain herbal supplements and alternative therapies were met with skepticism from regulatory bodies, who demanded extensive documentation and clinical trials before granting approval.

Undeterred, Dr. Wells immersed herself in the intricate world of research and documentation. She meticulously recorded every patient's progress, carefully noting the dosages, combinations, and outcomes of each natural treatment. With each successful case study, she built a compelling body of evidence to support her holistic approach.

"I understand the need for caution and oversight," she explained to a panel of skeptical regulators. "However, we must also recognize that the path to true healing often lies beyond the confines of conventional thinking. By embracing a more open-minded and integrative approach, we can unlock the full potential of nature's remedies while ensuring patient safety."

Through her unwavering commitment to her principles, Dr. Wells gradually gained allies within the medical community. Physicians and researchers who had initially been skeptical began to take notice of her work, intrigued by the positive outcomes they witnessed in her patients.

"I must admit, I was initially doubtful of your methods," confessed a respected endocrinologist during a chance encounter. "But the remarkable improvements I've seen in some of my patients who have sought your care have made me reconsider my stance. Perhaps there is wisdom in embracing a more holistic approach."

As the tide of resistance began to ebb, Dr. Wells remained steadfast in her mission. She understood that true change often came at a cost, and she was willing to weather the storms of skepticism and opposition. For her, staying true to her principles was not merely a choice but a calling – a commitment to explore the boundless potential of nature's healing powers and to offer hope to those who had been let down by conventional treatments.

With each patient she helped, with each small victory against the resistance, Dr. Wells's resolve grew stronger. She knew that her journey was far from over, but she also recognized that she was part of a larger movement – a paradigm shift towards a more integrative and compassionate approach to healthcare.

6.5: A Matter of Conviction

As the whispers of skepticism grew louder, Dr. Wells found herself at a crossroads. The conventional medical establishment, deeply entrenched in its ways, viewed her holistic approach with suspicion and disdain. Yet, she remained unwavering in her conviction, fueled by the remarkable transformations she witnessed in her patients.

The challenges came in waves, each one testing the depths of her resolve. Colleagues she once respected now regarded her as a misguided idealist, peddling unproven remedies. Their dismissive attitudes stung, but Dr. Wells refused to let their doubts diminish her belief in the power of natural healing.

One particularly heated encounter etched itself into her memory. During a medical conference, she had been invited to present her findings on the efficacy of herbal supplements in managing thyroid disorders. As she took the stage, the atmosphere was thick with skepticism, and she could sense the audience's collective eye-roll.

Undeterred, Dr. Wells launched into her presentation, meticulously detailing the scientific evidence and case studies that supported her approach. She spoke with passion, her words carrying the weight of her unwavering belief in the profound healing potential of nature.

As she delved deeper into her research, the murmurs of dissent grew louder. Skeptics fired off questions, their voices laced with condescension, challenging the validity of her methods and the credibility of her sources.

But Dr. Wells stood her ground, her conviction unshakable. She countered each objection with calm, reasoned responses, backed by a wealth of data and personal experiences. Her patients' remarkable journeys were her strongest allies, living proof that her unconventional approach yielded tangible results.

The confrontation escalated, with tempers flaring on both sides. Dr. Wells could feel the weight of the establishment's resistance pressing down upon her, but she refused to yield. This was more than just a battle of ideologies; it was a fight for the right to explore alternative paths to healing, to challenge the status quo, and to offer hope to those who had been failed by traditional methods.

As the debate raged on, a hush fell over the room when a soft voice rose from the back. It belonged to a woman who had been one of Dr. Wells's earliest patients, a woman who had once been bedridden by the debilitating effects of hypothyroidism.

With tears in her eyes, she recounted her journey from despair to renewed vitality, crediting Dr. Wells's holistic approach for her remarkable recovery. Her testimony was a powerful reminder of the human lives at stake, the individuals whose well-being transcended academic debates and institutional politics.

In that moment, the atmosphere shifted, and a glimmer of understanding flickered across the faces of some of the skeptics. While the resistance remained formidable, a seed of doubt had been planted, a crack in the foundation of rigid beliefs.

As Dr. Wells left the conference, her resolve fortified, she knew that the path ahead would be fraught with challenges. But she also knew that her conviction was unshakable, her belief in the transformative power of natural healing unwavering.

This was not a battle to be won through force or aggression but through perseverance, compassion, and an unwavering commitment to the well-being of her patients. Each triumph, no matter how small, would be a stepping stone toward a greater understanding and acceptance of integrative healthcare.

Dr. Wells's conviction was not born of arrogance or a desire for recognition; it stemmed from a deep-rooted belief that there were alternative paths to healing, paths that had been overlooked or dismissed by the conventional medical establishment. Her mission was to explore these avenues, to uncover the wisdom of ancient traditions, and to integrate them with modern scientific knowledge, creating a holistic approach that addressed the body, mind, and spirit.

As she looked to the future, Dr. Wells knew that the road ahead would be paved with obstacles, but she was prepared to face them head-on. Her conviction was her compass, guiding her through the storms of skepticism and resistance, ever-focused on the goal of offering hope and healing to those who sought it.

For Dr. Wells, this was not merely a career; it was a calling, a sacred duty to alleviate suffering and empower individuals to reclaim their health and vitality. With each step forward, she carried the weight of her patients' trust, a responsibility she embraced with humility and unwavering determination.

The resistance might be formidable, but Dr. Wells's conviction burned brighter than ever, a beacon of hope in a world that often overlooked the healing power of nature. And with each patient whose life was transformed, her resolve only grew stronger, fueling her journey towards a paradigm shift in healthcare, one that embraced the wisdom of the past and the promise of the future.

Chapter 7: Ripples of Change

7.1 Inspiring Others

As Dr. Sarah Wells' pioneering work in holistic thyroid care gained momentum, she found herself at the forefront of a burgeoning movement. Her unwavering dedication to natural healing and her remarkable success stories inspired others to question the conventional approach to hypothyroidism.

One such individual was Emily Thompson, a young woman who had been struggling with thyroid issues for years. Despite faithfully following her doctor's prescribed synthetic medication regimen, Emily's symptoms persisted, leaving her exhausted, overweight, and emotionally drained.

It was during a chance encounter at a local health food store that Emily first learned about Dr. Wells' clinic. Intrigued by the concept of natural remedies, she decided to make an appointment, her skepticism tempered by a glimmer of hope.

Emily's initial consultation with Dr. Wells was a revelation. For the first time, she felt truly heard and understood. Dr. Wells took the time to listen to her story, delving into the intricate details of her symptoms and lifestyle. She explained the holistic approach, emphasizing the importance of addressing the root causes of thyroid imbalance rather than merely masking the symptoms.

Under Dr. Wells' guidance, Emily embarked on a transformative journey. She adopted a thyroid-friendly diet rich in nutrient-dense foods, incorporated herbal supplements, and practiced stress-reduction techniques like meditation and gentle yoga. Slowly but surely, her energy levels began to rise, her mood improved, and the stubborn weight started to melt away.

Emily's remarkable transformation inspired her friends and family to explore natural healing methods for their own health concerns. Word of Dr. Wells' clinic spread like wildfire, attracting individuals from all walks of life who had grown disillusioned with the limitations of conventional medicine.

Among them was a retired schoolteacher named Martha, who had been battling hypothyroidism for decades. Despite her unwavering compliance with her prescribed medication, Martha's symptoms had only worsened over time, leaving her feeling like a mere shadow of her former vibrant self.

Encouraged by Emily's success story, Martha decided to give Dr. Wells' approach a try. She was immediately struck by the warmth and compassion of the clinic's staff, who treated her not just as a patient but as a whole person deserving of individualized care.

Under Dr. Wells' guidance, Martha embarked on a journey of self-discovery, learning to listen to her body's innate wisdom and embrace a holistic lifestyle. Through dietary changes, herbal remedies, and mindfulness practices, she gradually regained her energy, clarity of mind, and zest for life.

Martha's transformation was so profound that her children and grandchildren took notice. Inspired by her newfound vitality, they too began to explore natural healing modalities, seeking out practitioners who could guide them on their own paths to wellness.

As the ripples of change spread outward, Dr. Wells found herself at the center of a growing community of individuals united by a shared commitment to holistic health. Her clinic became a hub of knowledge and support, attracting not only patients but also aspiring practitioners eager to learn from her pioneering work.

Among them was a young medical student named Alex, who had grown disillusioned with the reductionist approach to healthcare taught in his classes. Drawn to Dr. Wells' integrative philosophy, he began volunteering at the clinic, eager to learn from her wealth of experience.

Under Dr. Wells' mentorship, Alex discovered a whole new world of healing modalities that had been largely overlooked in his formal training. He witnessed firsthand the transformative power of natural remedies, dietary interventions, and mind-body practices in restoring balance and vitality.

Inspired by the profound impact he saw on the lives of patients, Alex made a pivotal decision: he would dedicate his career to bridging the gap between conventional and holistic medicine, becoming a catalyst for change within the healthcare system.

As word of Dr. Wells' groundbreaking work spread, she found herself inundated with requests for speaking engagements, media interviews, and collaborations with like-minded practitioners from around the world. Her message of empowerment and natural healing resonated deeply with those who had grown weary of the one-size-fits-all approach to healthcare.

Through her tireless efforts, Dr. Wells became a beacon of hope for countless individuals seeking a more holistic and personalized approach to thyroid care. Her unwavering commitment to challenging the status quo and embracing the wisdom of nature inspired a ripple effect that would forever change the landscape of healthcare.

7.2 Challenging the Status Quo

As Dr. Wells' integrative approach to treating hypothyroidism gained traction, she found herself at the forefront of a burgeoning movement challenging the status quo of conventional medicine. Her unwavering commitment to holistic healing resonated with patients and practitioners alike, inspiring them to question long-held beliefs and embrace a more comprehensive understanding of health and wellness.

One such individual was Dr. Michael Ramirez, a seasoned endocrinologist who had spent decades prescribing synthetic thyroid medications to his patients. Despite his initial skepticism, Dr. Ramirez couldn't ignore the remarkable improvements he witnessed in those who had embraced Dr. Wells' natural remedies.

"I'll be honest, when I first heard about Dr. Wells' methods, I was dismissive," Dr. Ramirez admitted during a medical conference. "As a specialist in endocrinology, I had been trained to rely solely on pharmaceutical interventions. The idea of using herbs, dietary changes, and ancient healing practices seemed like a step backwards."

However, Dr. Ramirez's perspective began to shift when one of his long-time patients, Sarah Thompson, returned to his office with a newfound vitality. Sarah had been struggling with hypothyroidism for years, and despite being on the highest dosage of synthetic thyroid medication, her symptoms persisted.

"I was at my wit's end," Sarah recalled. "I felt like a shell of my former self – constantly fatigued, battling weight gain, and struggling with brain fog. That's when a friend recommended Dr. Wells' clinic."

Sarah's experience with Dr. Wells' integrative approach was nothing short of transformative. Through a combination of herbal supplements, acupuncture, and dietary modifications, her energy levels soared, her weight stabilized, and her mental clarity returned.

"When Sarah walked into my office, I couldn't believe the change," Dr. Ramirez marveled. "She was radiant, vibrant, and full of life – a far cry from the exhausted, discouraged woman I had seen just months earlier."

Intrigued by Sarah's remarkable recovery, Dr. Ramirez began to delve into the research behind Dr. Wells' methods. What he discovered challenged his long-held beliefs about the treatment of hypothyroidism.

"I realized that the conventional approach, while effective for some, was far from a one-size-fits-all solution," he explained. "By incorporating natural remedies and addressing the underlying imbalances, Dr. Wells was able to provide a more holistic and personalized approach to healing."

Inspired by these findings, Dr. Ramirez began to integrate elements of Dr. Wells' approach into his own practice. He encouraged his patients to explore dietary changes, recommended herbal supplements, and even referred some to Dr. Wells' clinic for acupuncture and stress-reduction techniques.

The results were undeniable. Patients who had previously struggled with persistent symptoms found relief, and those who had been resistant to conventional treatments experienced newfound vitality.

"It was a humbling experience," Dr. Ramirez admitted. "I had to let go of my preconceived notions and embrace a more open-minded approach to healing. By combining the best of conventional and holistic medicine, we were able to provide our patients with truly comprehensive care."

Dr. Ramirez's journey from skeptic to advocate was not an isolated case. As word of Dr. Wells' success spread, more and more healthcare professionals began to take notice. Some were initially drawn by curiosity, while others sought alternative solutions for their patients who had failed to respond to traditional treatments.

Gradually, a community of like-minded practitioners emerged, united in their desire to challenge the status quo and explore the potential of integrative medicine. They formed study groups, attended conferences, and shared their experiences, each contributing to a growing body of knowledge and best practices.

"It's a paradigm shift that's long overdue," remarked Dr. Samantha Lee, a naturopathic physician who had been collaborating with Dr. Wells. "For too long, we've been operating within silos, ignoring the interconnectedness of the body, mind, and spirit. By embracing a holistic approach, we're able to treat the whole person, not just their symptoms."

As this movement gained momentum, it began to ripple outward, challenging the very foundations of the healthcare system. Patients became more informed and empowered, demanding a greater emphasis on preventative care and personalized treatment plans. Medical schools started to incorporate courses on integrative medicine, recognizing the need to train future practitioners in a more comprehensive approach.

While the road ahead was not without its challenges, Dr. Wells and her allies remained steadfast in their commitment to transforming the landscape of healthcare. They understood that true healing required a willingness to question the status quo and embrace new perspectives, even in the face of resistance and skepticism.

"Change is never easy," Dr. Wells acknowledged. "But when we open our minds to the possibilities, we unlock the true potential of healing – a potential that lies not only in modern medicine but also in the wisdom of nature and the resilience of the human spirit."

With each patient who found relief, each practitioner who embraced a more integrative approach, and each institution that acknowledged the value of holistic healing, the ripples of change grew stronger, paving the way for a new era of healthcare – one that honored the body's innate wisdom and celebrated the power of nature's thyroid solution.

7.3 A Growing Movement

As Dr. Wells' pioneering work in integrative thyroid care gained traction, a ripple effect began to spread throughout the medical community. Her unwavering commitment to holistic healing and natural remedies inspired others to question the status quo and explore alternative approaches to wellness.

One such individual was Dr. Emily Nguyen, a young endocrinologist fresh out of residency. Disillusioned by the one-size-fits-all approach to thyroid disorders she had witnessed during her training, Dr. Nguyen found herself drawn to Dr. Wells' work. She attended a seminar hosted by the naturopathic clinic, where she was exposed to the transformative power of integrative medicine.

"It was like a veil had been lifted from my eyes," Dr. Nguyen recalled. "I had been taught to treat hypothyroidism with synthetic hormones and little else. But Dr. Wells showed me that there was so much more we could do to address the root causes and support the body's natural healing processes."

Inspired by this newfound perspective, Dr. Nguyen began incorporating elements of holistic care into her practice. She encouraged her patients to make dietary changes, explore stress-reduction techniques, and consider herbal supplements alongside conventional treatments. The results were remarkable, with many patients reporting significant improvements in their energy levels, weight management, and overall well-being.

Word of Dr. Nguyen's success spread quickly, and soon other healthcare professionals began to take notice. Physicians, nurses, and therapists from various disciplines sought out Dr. Wells' guidance, eager to learn more about integrative thyroid care.

One such individual was Dr. Marcus Alvarez, a respected family physician with a thriving practice. Initially skeptical of Dr. Wells' unconventional methods, Dr. Alvarez found himself intrigued after witnessing the remarkable recovery of one of his long-time patients, who had struggled with hypothyroidism for years.

"I couldn't believe the transformation," Dr. Alvarez admitted. "This patient had tried every conventional treatment under the sun, but nothing seemed to work. Then, after following Dr. Wells' recommendations, she was like a different person – full of energy, her weight stabilized, and her mood improved dramatically."

Driven by curiosity and a desire to better serve his patients, Dr. Alvarez reached out to Dr. Wells, and the two formed an unlikely partnership. Together, they began to collaborate on developing comprehensive treatment plans that combined the best of conventional and holistic medicine.

As the movement gained momentum, a network of like-minded healthcare professionals emerged, united by a shared vision of integrative thyroid care. They organized conferences, workshops, and online forums, fostering a vibrant community dedicated to exploring natural solutions and challenging the boundaries of traditional medicine.

One such event was the annual "Thyroid Wellness Summit," which brought together experts from around the world to share their insights and experiences. Attendees had the opportunity to learn about cutting-edge research, participate in hands-on workshops, and connect with others who shared their passion for holistic healing.

"It's incredible to see how far we've come," Dr. Wells remarked during the summit's opening address. "Just a few years ago, I was a lone voice in the wilderness, fighting an uphill battle against the medical establishment. But now, we are a growing movement, united in our commitment to providing comprehensive, patient-centered care for those struggling with thyroid disorders."

As the movement gained traction, it began to attract the attention of researchers and academics. Universities and medical centers launched studies to investigate the efficacy of integrative approaches to thyroid care, lending scientific credibility to the work pioneered by Dr. Wells and her colleagues.

The ripples of change were undeniable, and the once-marginalized field of holistic thyroid care was rapidly gaining mainstream acceptance. Patients were empowered to take an active role in their healing journeys, and healthcare professionals were embracing a more holistic, personalized approach to treatment.

While challenges and skepticism remained, the growing movement was a testament to the power of perseverance, innovation, and a unwavering belief in the healing potential of nature. As Dr. Wells looked to the future, she felt a sense of hope and gratitude, knowing that her pioneering work had paved the way for a new era of integrative healthcare.

7.4 Embracing Diversity

As Dr. Wells's integrative approach to treating hypothyroidism gained traction, she witnessed a remarkable phenomenon – people from all walks of life began to embrace the principles of holistic healing. Her clinic became a sanctuary for individuals seeking alternative paths to wellness, transcending boundaries of age, ethnicity, and socioeconomic status.

One of the first to join Dr. Wells's growing community was Amara, a young woman in her late twenties. Amara had been struggling with hypothyroidism since her teenage years, and despite being on conventional medication, her symptoms persisted. She felt lethargic, her hair was thinning, and she struggled with weight fluctuations. When she stumbled upon Dr. Wells's clinic, she was initially skeptical but decided to give it a chance.

"I had tried everything, and nothing seemed to work," Amara recalled. "But the moment I stepped into Dr. Wells's clinic, I felt a sense of hope that I hadn't experienced in years."

Under Dr. Wells's guidance, Amara embarked on a holistic journey that involved dietary changes, herbal supplements, and mindfulness practices. Within a few months, her energy levels soared, her hair regained its luster, and her weight stabilized. Amara became a vocal advocate for integrative medicine, sharing her story with others and inspiring them to explore alternative healing paths.

Another patient who found solace in Dr. Wells's approach was Miguel, a retired construction worker in his sixties. Miguel had been diagnosed with hypothyroidism after years of unexplained fatigue and muscle aches. His condition had taken a toll on his physical and mental well-being, and he struggled to find joy in the activities he once loved.

"I felt like I was losing myself," Miguel admitted. "I couldn't keep up with my grandkids, and even simple tasks seemed like a monumental effort."

Desperate for relief, Miguel sought out Dr. Wells's clinic. Through a combination of acupuncture, herbal remedies, and stress-reduction techniques, Miguel gradually regained his vitality. He marveled at the transformative power of nature and the ancient wisdom that had been overlooked by conventional medicine.

"It's like I've been given a second chance at life," Miguel beamed. "I never imagined that something as simple as plants and needles could have such a profound impact."

As word of Dr. Wells's success spread, her clinic became a melting pot of individuals from diverse backgrounds, united by their desire for holistic healing. From busy professionals seeking respite from the stresses of modern life to stay-at-home parents yearning for renewed energy, the clinic's doors were open to all.

Dr. Wells embraced this diversity wholeheartedly, recognizing that each individual's journey was unique. She tailored her treatment plans to address the specific needs and circumstances of her patients, acknowledging the intricate interplay between physical, emotional, and spiritual well-being.

"Healing is not a one-size-fits-all approach," Dr. Wells would often say. "We must embrace the complexities of each individual's life and craft a path that resonates with their values and beliefs."

Through her unwavering commitment to inclusivity and personalized care, Dr. Wells fostered a community that celebrated the richness of human diversity. Her clinic became a sanctuary where people from all walks of life could find solace, support, and a renewed sense of hope.

As the ripples of change spread outward, Dr. Wells's integrative approach inspired others to question the limitations of conventional medicine and explore the vast potential of holistic healing. Her work not only transformed the lives of her patients but also challenged the boundaries of mainstream healthcare, paving the way for a more inclusive and compassionate approach to wellness.

7.5 Paving the Way

As Dr. Wells' integrative approach to treating hypothyroidism gained traction, her work began paving the way for a broader acceptance of holistic wellness practices. Her unwavering dedication to exploring natural remedies and challenging the conventional medical paradigm inspired others to question the status quo and seek alternative paths to healing.

The ripples of change extended far beyond the walls of her clinic. Patients who had experienced remarkable improvements in their health became ambassadors for Dr. Wells' methods, sharing their stories with friends, family, and communities. Word spread rapidly, and soon, people from all walks of life sought her guidance, eager to embrace a more holistic approach to their well-being.

One such individual was Emily, a young mother who had struggled with hypothyroidism for years. After trying countless medications and enduring their debilitating side effects, she stumbled upon Dr. Wells' work and decided to give her integrative approach a chance. Within weeks of implementing the dietary changes, herbal supplements, and stress-reduction techniques recommended by Dr. Wells, Emily's energy levels soared, and her mood improved dramatically.

"It was like emerging from a fog," Emily recalled. "For the first time in years, I felt alive again. Dr. Wells didn't just treat my thyroid condition; she helped me reclaim my life."

Inspired by her transformation, Emily became an advocate for Dr. Wells' work, sharing her story with local support groups and online communities. Her testimony resonated with countless others who had grown disillusioned with conventional treatments, igniting a spark of hope within them.

As the demand for Dr. Wells' services grew, she recognized the need to expand her reach and empower others to embrace holistic wellness. She began offering workshops and seminars, teaching healthcare professionals, students, and the general public about the principles of integrative medicine and the power of natural remedies.

One such seminar attendee was Dr. Marcus Nguyen, a young physician who had grown increasingly dissatisfied with the limitations of traditional medicine. "Dr. Wells' approach opened my eyes to a world of possibilities," he shared. "I realized that true healing extends beyond prescribing pills and addressing symptoms. It's about treating the whole person – mind, body, and spirit."

Inspired by Dr. Wells' teachings, Dr. Nguyen began incorporating holistic practices into his own practice, recommending dietary changes, stress-reduction techniques, and natural supplements to his patients. The positive results he witnessed were undeniable, and he soon became an advocate for integrative medicine within his medical community.

As the movement gained momentum, Dr. Wells found herself at the forefront of a paradigm shift in healthcare. Her pioneering work challenged long-held beliefs and paved the way for a more inclusive and comprehensive approach to wellness.

However, the path was not without obstacles. Skeptics and naysayers continued to question the validity of her methods, citing a lack of scientific evidence and adherence to traditional medical protocols. But Dr. Wells remained steadfast in her convictions, recognizing that true progress often requires challenging the status quo.

"We cannot allow fear of the unknown to hold us back," she proclaimed. "Nature has provided us with an abundance of healing resources, and it is our duty to explore and harness their potential for the betterment of humanity."

With each success story and each life transformed, Dr. Wells' work gained credibility and inspired others to join her mission. Slowly but surely, the barriers began to crumble, and a new era of integrative healthcare emerged, one that embraced the wisdom of ancient healing traditions while harnessing the power of modern science.

As Dr. Wells looked back on her journey, she felt a profound sense of gratitude for the countless individuals who had joined her in paving the way for this paradigm shift. From patients who had found renewed hope to healthcare professionals who had embraced a more holistic approach, each person played a vital role in shaping a future where wellness was not just a pursuit but a way of life.

With a renewed sense of purpose, Dr. Wells continued her work, determined to leave a lasting legacy – a world where the healing power of nature was celebrated, and true wellness was within reach for all.

Chapter 8: The Clinic's Heartbeat

8.1 A Sanctuary of Healing

In the heart of Metropolis, nestled amidst the towering skyscrapers and bustling streets, a sanctuary of healing emerged – Dr. Sarah Wells's integrative clinic for thyroid disorders. This haven stood as a beacon of hope for those seeking solace from the relentless grip of hypothyroidism, offering a holistic approach that celebrated the restorative power of nature.

As patients stepped through the doors, they were immediately enveloped in an atmosphere of tranquility. The soothing hues of the walls, adorned with vibrant murals depicting lush botanical gardens, created a sense of serenity that contrasted sharply with the frenetic pace of the city beyond. The air was infused with the gentle aromas of essential oils, each carefully selected for their therapeutic properties.

At the heart of the clinic's design was a central courtyard, a verdant oasis where the sound of a trickling fountain mingled with the melodic chirping of birds. Here, patients could find solace in nature's embrace, basking in the warmth of the sun or seeking refuge beneath the canopy of trees that swayed gently in the breeze. It was a space that fostered healing not only for the body but also for the mind and spirit.

The reception area, adorned with plush seating and warm lighting, welcomed patients with a sense of comfort and familiarity. The staff, trained in the art of compassionate care, greeted each individual with a genuine smile and a listening ear, ready to address their concerns and alleviate their anxieties.

Beyond the reception, a series of treatment rooms awaited, each meticulously designed to cater to the specific needs of the patients. In one room, the gentle hum of acupuncture needles harmonized with the soothing melodies of ambient music, guiding patients into a state of deep relaxation. Nearby, the aroma of freshly brewed herbal teas wafted from a cozy nook, where patients could consult with Dr. Wells and her team of naturopaths to discuss personalized treatment plans.

The clinic's apothecary was a treasure trove of natural remedies, housing an array of carefully curated herbs, tinctures, and supplements. Here, patients could explore the wealth of nature's bounty, guided by knowledgeable staff who took the time to educate and empower them on the path to wellness.

Throughout the clinic, every detail was thoughtfully curated to foster an environment that nurtured the body, mind, and spirit. From the soft lighting that mimicked the gentle glow of candlelight to the plush textiles that invited patients to sink into a state of tranquility, each element was designed to create a sanctuary where healing could flourish.

But the true essence of this sanctuary extended beyond its physical manifestation. It was a place where patients felt heard, understood, and supported on their journey towards reclaiming their vitality. Dr. Wells and her team approached each individual with compassion, recognizing the unique challenges they faced and tailoring their care to address their specific needs.

Within these walls, the conventional boundaries of medicine were transcended, and a new paradigm of holistic healing took root. It was a sanctuary where the ancient wisdom of nature intertwined with modern scientific understanding, where the art of listening was elevated to the same level as the science of treatment.

As patients left the clinic, their steps felt lighter, their spirits buoyed by a newfound sense of hope. For within this sanctuary, they had found not just a place of healing but a community that embraced them, a haven where their struggles were validated and their paths to wellness were illuminated by the radiant light of compassion and understanding.

8.2 Tailored Treatments

In the heart of Metropolis, nestled among towering skyscrapers and bustling streets, Dr. Sarah Wells's clinic stood as a sanctuary of healing.

Here, patients found solace in a holistic approach that celebrated the intricate dance between body, mind, and spirit. Each individual who walked through the doors was treated not merely as a case file but as a unique tapestry woven from countless threads of life experiences, emotions, and environmental influences.

Dr. Wells understood that no two patients were alike, and her approach reflected this fundamental truth. She embraced the art of tailoring treatments, meticulously crafting personalized plans that addressed the root causes of each patient's hypothyroidism. It was a delicate balance, a harmonious symphony of ancient wisdom and modern scientific understanding.

The clinic's reception area exuded a warm and welcoming ambiance, with natural elements seamlessly blending with modern design. Soft instrumental music filled the air, creating a soothing atmosphere that instantly put visitors at ease. Here, patients would embark on their journey towards holistic wellness, leaving behind the sterile confines of conventional medical facilities.

During the initial consultation, Dr. Wells would listen intently, her empathetic gaze encouraging patients to share their stories without reservation. She understood that the path to healing often began with the simple act of being heard, of having one's struggles acknowledged and validated.

With each patient's unique narrative in mind, Dr. Wells would carefully curate a comprehensive treatment plan. For some, dietary modifications were the cornerstone, incorporating nutrient-rich whole foods and eliminating inflammatory triggers. Others found solace in the ancient art of acupuncture, where the strategic placement of needles along energy meridians restored balance and harmony.

Herbal remedies played a pivotal role in many treatment plans, drawing upon nature's bountiful offerings. Dr. Wells meticulously researched and sourced high-quality botanical extracts, each chosen for its specific therapeutic properties. From adaptogenic herbs that supported the body's stress response to gentle thyroid-nourishing blends, these natural allies worked in synergy to restore equilibrium.

Stress management techniques were also woven into the tapestry of care, recognizing the profound impact of emotional well-being on physical health. Patients were guided through mindfulness practices, breathing exercises, and gentle yoga sequences, empowering them to cultivate inner peace and resilience.

Throughout the healing journey, Dr. Wells remained a steadfast companion, adjusting and refining the treatment plans as needed. She celebrated each milestone, no matter how small, and encouraged her patients to embrace a holistic lifestyle that nurtured their overall well-being.

One such patient, Emily, had struggled with hypothyroidism for years, her energy levels plummeting and her once-vibrant spirit dimming. Under Dr. Wells's guidance, Emily embarked on a transformative path. Through a carefully curated blend of dietary changes, herbal supplements, and mindfulness practices, she gradually regained her vitality. The once-daunting task of climbing a flight of stairs became effortless, and her radiant smile returned, a testament to the power of holistic healing.

Another patient, Michael, had grappled with stubborn weight gain and brain fog, hindering his ability to excel in his career. Dr. Wells's integrative approach addressed the underlying imbalances, incorporating acupuncture sessions to restore energy flow and targeted herbal formulas to support thyroid function. Slowly but surely, the fog lifted, and Michael's mental clarity returned, allowing him to thrive both personally and professionally.

Each success story added another thread to the tapestry of healing that adorned the clinic's walls. Patients shared their journeys, inspiring others to embrace the transformative power of nature and holistic living. The clinic became a beacon of hope, a sanctuary where individuals could reclaim their health and rediscover the joy of living life to its fullest potential.

As Dr. Wells walked the halls, she couldn't help but feel a profound sense of gratitude for the opportunity to make a difference in so many lives. Her unwavering dedication to holistic healing had blossomed into a thriving practice, a testament to the resilience of the human spirit and the profound wisdom found in nature's embrace.

8.3 Nurturing Connections

In the heart of Metropolis, Dr. Sarah Wells's clinic stood as a beacon of hope for those seeking solace from the relentless grip of hypothyroidism. Beyond the walls of this sanctuary, a vibrant community had blossomed, nurtured by the shared experiences and unwavering support of its members.

As patients stepped through the doors, they were enveloped in a warm embrace of understanding and camaraderie. The waiting room buzzed with the gentle murmur of conversations, where stories of struggle and triumph were exchanged freely. Here, they found solace in the knowledge that they were not alone in their journey.

Dr. Wells believed that healing extended beyond the physical realm, encompassing the emotional and spiritual aspects of one's being. She encouraged her patients to forge connections, to lean on each other for support, and to draw strength from the collective resilience of the community.

One such patient, Emily, had been battling hypothyroidism for years, her once vibrant spirit dimmed by the relentless fatigue and emotional turmoil that accompanied the condition. Upon her first visit to the clinic, she was greeted by a group of women who had walked a similar path. Their shared experiences and empathy immediately put her at ease, and she found herself opening up in ways she never thought possible.

As Emily embarked on her holistic treatment plan, she found solace in the weekly support group meetings facilitated by Dr. Wells. Here, they delved into the intricacies of their conditions, shared coping strategies, and celebrated even the smallest victories. The bonds forged within these sessions transcended the boundaries of patient and practitioner, blossoming into genuine friendships.

One such friend was Sarah, a young mother who had struggled with hypothyroidism since the birth of her first child. The weight gain and emotional upheaval had taken a toll on her self-confidence, and she found herself withdrawing from the world. At the clinic, however, she discovered a safe haven where she could be her authentic self, surrounded by individuals who understood her plight.

Together, Emily and Sarah navigated the ups and downs of their healing journeys, leaning on each other for support and encouragement. They celebrated milestones together, whether it was shedding a few pounds or regaining the energy to chase after their children. Their shared laughter and tears forged an unbreakable bond, a testament to the power of human connection in the face of adversity.

Dr. Wells recognized the profound impact these connections had on her patients' overall well-being. She encouraged them to participate in group activities, such as gentle yoga sessions or nature walks, where they could connect with themselves, with nature, and with one another. These shared experiences fostered a sense of community and belonging, reminding them that they were not alone on this journey.

The clinic's walls echoed with the laughter and camaraderie that flourished within its embrace. Patients who had once felt isolated and misunderstood found solace in the understanding and empathy of their peers. They celebrated each other's triumphs, lifted one another during moments of struggle, and formed lasting bonds that extended far beyond the confines of the clinic.

As the community grew stronger, so too did the collective voice advocating for holistic approaches to thyroid care. Patients became ambassadors, sharing their stories and inspiring others to explore alternative paths to healing. Their resilience and unwavering support for one another served as a powerful testament to the transformative power of human connection in the face of adversity.

In the heart of Dr. Wells's clinic, a tapestry of hope and healing was woven, thread by thread, through the shared experiences and unwavering support of its members. It was a sanctuary where connections blossomed, spirits were uplifted, and the journey towards wellness was embraced with open arms and open hearts.

8.4 Celebrating Milestones

As the months and years passed, Dr. Wells's clinic became a sanctuary of hope for countless individuals seeking relief from the debilitating effects of hypothyroidism. Each patient's journey was a testament to the power of holistic healing, and their milestones were celebrated with great joy and gratitude.

The clinic's walls echoed with stories of transformation, serving as a constant reminder of the profound impact of Dr. Wells's integrative approach. From the moment patients stepped through the doors, they were enveloped in an atmosphere of warmth and compassion, where their struggles were understood and their triumphs were cherished.

One such patient was Emily, a young mother who had been struggling with hypothyroidism for years. Her fatigue had become so overwhelming that she could barely keep up with the demands of daily life, let alone enjoy precious moments with her children. After months of following Dr. Wells's personalized treatment plan, which included dietary changes, herbal supplements, and mindfulness practices, Emily's energy levels soared, and her zest for life returned.

The clinic celebrated Emily's milestone with a heartwarming gathering, where she shared her journey and expressed her profound gratitude for the support she received. Her radiant smile and vibrant energy were a stark contrast to the exhausted woman who had first walked through the doors, and her story inspired others to embrace the transformative power of holistic healing.

Another patient, Michael, had grappled with the emotional turmoil that often accompanied hypothyroidism. His mood swings and bouts of depression had strained his relationships and left him feeling isolated. Through a combination of acupuncture, herbal remedies, and counseling, Michael gradually regained emotional equilibrium. His milestone was marked by a heartfelt letter he wrote to Dr. Wells, expressing his gratitude for helping him reclaim his sense of self and reconnect with those he loved.

As the clinic's reputation grew, patients from far and wide sought its services, each with their own unique story and set of challenges. Dr. Wells and her team embraced these diverse journeys, tailoring their approach to meet the individual needs of every patient. Whether it was a young athlete struggling with weight gain, a busy executive battling brain fog, or an elderly woman seeking relief from hair loss, the clinic's doors were open, offering a beacon of hope and healing.

Milestones were celebrated in myriad ways, from intimate gatherings where patients shared their triumphs to larger events that brought the community together. Artwork adorned the clinic's walls, depicting the transformative power of nature's remedies, and a garden bloomed with herbs and flowers, serving as a reminder of the healing potential that surrounded them.

Each celebration was a testament to the resilience of the human spirit and the unwavering commitment of Dr. Wells and her team. They had defied the odds, challenged the status quo, and paved the way for a new era of integrative healthcare, where the wisdom of ancient traditions and the advancements of modern science converged to offer comprehensive and compassionate care.

As the sun set on another day at the clinic, Dr. Wells would often pause to reflect on the countless lives that had been touched by her work. She felt a profound sense of gratitude for the opportunity to make a difference and a renewed determination to continue pushing boundaries and inspiring others to embrace the healing power of nature's thyroid solution.

8.5 A Beacon of Hope

As the sun's golden rays filtered through the large windows of the clinic, Dr. Sarah Wells couldn't help but feel a sense of pride and fulfillment. This sanctuary, born from her unwavering determination and belief in the power of natural healing, had become a beacon of hope for countless individuals seeking relief from the debilitating effects of hypothyroidism.

The clinic's walls, adorned with vibrant murals depicting the beauty of nature, radiated a warm and welcoming energy. Each room was meticulously designed to create an atmosphere of tranquility, where patients could shed the weight of their burdens and embrace the healing journey ahead.

At the heart of this haven was a dedicated team of professionals, united by their shared passion for integrative care. From the gentle touch of the acupuncturists to the soothing voices of the counselors, every member played a vital role in nurturing the mind, body, and spirit of those who sought their guidance.

One such individual was Emily, a young woman who had struggled with hypothyroidism for years. Her journey had been a rollercoaster of emotions, marked by fatigue, weight fluctuations, and a constant sense of disconnection from her own body. Conventional treatments had offered little relief, leaving her feeling hopeless and alone.

But then, she found Dr. Wells's clinic.

From the moment Emily stepped through the doors, she felt a weight lifted from her shoulders. The compassionate staff listened intently to her story, acknowledging her struggles and validating her experiences. Together, they crafted a personalized treatment plan that combined dietary modifications, herbal supplements, and mindfulness practices.

Slowly but surely, Emily began to regain her vitality. The fog of fatigue lifted, and her energy levels soared. The once-stubborn pounds melted away, revealing a newfound confidence in her physical form. But perhaps most importantly, Emily's emotional well-being blossomed, as she learned to embrace self-care and cultivate inner peace.

Emily's transformation was just one of countless stories that unfolded within the walls of the clinic. Each patient's journey was unique, but they all shared a common thread – the unwavering belief that healing was possible, and that nature held the key to unlocking their full potential.

As word of the clinic's success spread, more and more individuals sought its guidance. Some came with trepidation, skeptical of the unconventional approaches but desperate for relief. Others arrived with open hearts and minds, eager to embrace a holistic path to wellness.

Regardless of their backgrounds or preconceptions, all were welcomed with open arms and treated with the utmost respect and compassion. Dr. Wells and her team understood that healing was a deeply personal journey, and they tailored their approach to meet the unique needs of each individual.

The clinic's impact extended far beyond its physical walls. Through educational outreach programs, workshops, and online resources, Dr. Wells and her colleagues shared their knowledge and insights with the broader community. They challenged long-held beliefs, sparked discussions, and inspired others to explore the vast potential of natural healing.

As the sun set over the clinic, casting warm hues across the peaceful gardens, Dr. Wells would often pause and reflect on the remarkable journey that had led her to this point. The seed of doubt that had once taken root within her had blossomed into a flourishing movement, empowering individuals to reclaim their health and embrace a holistic approach to wellness.

In that moment, she knew that her clinic was more than just a place of healing – it was a beacon of hope, shining a light on the path towards a future where integrative care was not just accepted but celebrated. And with each life transformed, that beacon burned brighter, illuminating the way for countless others seeking solace in nature's embrace.

Chapter 9: Confronting Adversity

9.1 Scrutiny Intensifies

As Dr. Sarah Wells' holistic approach to treating hypothyroidism gained traction, her clinic became a beacon of hope for countless individuals seeking relief from the debilitating symptoms of this condition. However, her unconventional methods also drew the attention of the medical establishment, and the scrutiny she faced began to intensify.

The first rumblings of discontent came from within the medical community itself. Colleagues who had once respected her work now regarded her with skepticism, questioning the validity of her natural remedies and the efficacy of her integrative approach. Whispers of "quackery" and "pseudoscience" echoed through the halls of hospitals and medical conferences.

Dr. Wells found herself on the defensive, forced to justify her methods time and again. She meticulously documented each patient's progress, compiling data that demonstrated the remarkable improvements achieved through her holistic treatments. Yet, the resistance remained steadfast, fueled by a deep-rooted belief in the superiority of conventional medicine.

The scrutiny extended beyond the medical realm, as regulatory bodies began to take notice of Dr. Wells' unconventional practices. Inspectors arrived unannounced at her clinic, scrutinizing every aspect of her operation with a critical eye. They pored over patient records, questioned her staff, and demanded explanations for her treatment protocols.

Undeterred, Dr. Wells welcomed these inspections as an opportunity to educate and dispel misconceptions. She opened her doors wide, inviting the inspectors to witness firsthand the transformative power of her holistic approach. With unwavering confidence, she walked them through her methodologies, citing scientific studies and drawing upon her extensive knowledge of natural remedies.

Yet, the scrutiny persisted, fueled by a deep-rooted skepticism and a fear of the unknown. Regulatory bodies raised concerns about the safety and efficacy of her treatments, questioning the validity of her research and the qualifications of her staff.

In the face of mounting pressure, Dr. Wells found herself navigating a complex web of bureaucracy and red tape. She spent countless hours poring over regulations, seeking legal counsel, and attending hearings to defend her practice. The emotional toll was immense, but her resolve remained unshaken.

Despite the challenges, Dr. Wells refused to compromise her principles or abandon her mission. She understood that true progress often comes at a cost, and she was willing to weather the storm in order to pave the way for a new era of integrative healthcare.

As the scrutiny intensified, Dr. Wells found solace in the unwavering support of her patients. Their testimonials of healing and renewed vitality served as a constant reminder of the profound impact her work had on their lives. These stories became her armor, shielding her from the doubts and criticisms that threatened to undermine her efforts.

With each inspection, each hearing, and each challenge, Dr. Wells emerged stronger and more determined than ever before. She recognized that the scrutiny she faced was not merely a personal battle but a larger struggle to reshape the landscape of healthcare, to embrace a more holistic and compassionate approach to healing.

9.2 Battling Bureaucracy

As Dr. Sarah Wells' holistic approach to treating hypothyroidism gained traction, the resistance from the medical establishment intensified. The bureaucratic machinery, deeply entrenched in traditional practices, viewed her methods as a threat to the status quo. The battle lines were drawn, and Dr. Wells found herself navigating a complex web of regulations and institutional barriers.

The first challenge arose when the state medical board received complaints from several conventional physicians, questioning the legitimacy of Dr. Wells' treatments. They argued that her reliance on natural remedies and alternative therapies lacked scientific evidence and could potentially put patients at risk.

Summoned to a hearing, Dr. Wells stood before a panel of stern-faced officials, each representing different facets of the medical establishment. Their skepticism was palpable, and their questions probed the very foundation of her work.

"Dr. Wells, can you provide us with peer-reviewed studies that validate the efficacy of your herbal supplements?" one panel member inquired, his tone laced with doubt.

Dr. Wells took a deep breath, steadying herself for the challenge ahead. "While there is a need for more research in this area, numerous traditional healing systems have relied on the power of plants for centuries," she began. "We cannot disregard the wealth of anecdotal evidence and the positive outcomes experienced by my patients."

The panel members exchanged glances, their expressions revealing a deep-rooted skepticism toward anything that strayed from conventional medicine.

"But how can we trust anecdotal evidence over rigorous clinical trials?" another panelist challenged. "Your methods lack the scientific rigor we demand in the medical field."

Dr. Wells understood their concerns, but she also recognized the limitations of a system that often dismissed alternative approaches without truly understanding them. "I acknowledge the importance of scientific validation," she responded calmly. "However, we must also remain open to exploring new avenues of healing, especially when traditional methods fail to provide lasting relief for many patients."

The hearing stretched on for hours, with Dr. Wells meticulously defending her practices and presenting case studies of patients who had experienced remarkable improvements under her care. She emphasized the importance of a holistic approach, addressing not only the physical symptoms but also the emotional and spiritual aspects of healing.

Despite her compelling arguments, the panel remained skeptical, bound by the rigid confines of conventional medicine. They expressed concerns about the potential risks associated with herbal remedies and the lack of standardization in their preparation and dosing.

Undeterred, Dr. Wells continued to advocate for her patients' right to explore alternative treatment options. She highlighted the growing body of research supporting the efficacy of certain natural remedies and the need for a more integrative approach to healthcare.

The battle extended beyond the confines of the hearing room, as Dr. Wells found herself navigating a labyrinth of bureaucratic hurdles. Obtaining licenses and certifications for her clinic became an uphill battle, with each step met with resistance from regulatory bodies deeply entrenched in traditional practices.

Determined to overcome these obstacles, Dr. Wells sought legal counsel and formed alliances with like-minded professionals. Together, they worked tirelessly to navigate the complex web of regulations, advocating for greater recognition and acceptance of integrative medicine.

The journey was arduous, but Dr. Wells remained steadfast in her conviction. She understood that true change often comes at a cost, and she was willing to weather the storm to pave the way for a more holistic approach to healthcare.

As the battle raged on, Dr. Wells found solace in the testimonies of her patients, whose lives had been transformed by her treatments. Their stories of renewed vitality and improved well-being fueled her determination to continue fighting for their right to access alternative healing modalities.

With each obstacle she overcame, Dr. Wells gained strength and resolve. She recognized that her battle was not just for herself or her clinic, but for the countless individuals seeking relief from the limitations of conventional medicine. Her unwavering spirit and commitment to her patients' well-being became a beacon of hope in the face of bureaucratic resistance.

9.3 Weathering the Storm

As Dr. Sarah Wells' holistic approach to treating hypothyroidism gained traction, the scrutiny from the medical establishment intensified. The conventional medical community, deeply entrenched in its ways, viewed her methods as a threat to the status quo. Their resistance manifested in various forms, from subtle undermining to outright opposition.

Despite the mounting pressure, Dr. Wells remained steadfast in her conviction. She understood that challenging long-held beliefs and practices would inevitably invite resistance, but she was prepared to weather the storm. Her unwavering dedication to her patients' well-being and her belief in the power of natural healing fueled her determination.

One of the most significant challenges Dr. Wells faced was the constant questioning of her credentials and qualifications. Critics argued that her naturopathic background and unconventional approach lacked the scientific rigor and evidence-based foundation that conventional medicine demanded. They dismissed her methods as unproven and potentially dangerous, citing a lack of large-scale clinical trials and peer-reviewed research.

However, Dr. Wells was not deterred. She meticulously documented her patients' progress, carefully tracking their symptoms, lab results, and overall well-being. The overwhelmingly positive outcomes spoke volumes, serving as a testament to the efficacy of her holistic approach. With each success story, she gained more confidence and resolve to continue her mission.

The resistance also manifested in the form of bureaucratic hurdles and regulatory challenges. Certain governing bodies questioned the legality of her practices, citing concerns over the use of herbal supplements and alternative therapies. Dr. Wells found herself navigating a complex web of regulations, often feeling like she was swimming against the current.

Undaunted, she sought legal counsel and collaborated with like-minded professionals to ensure compliance with all relevant laws and guidelines. She attended countless meetings, presented her case with unwavering conviction, and fought tirelessly to maintain the integrity of her clinic and the services she provided.

Throughout this turbulent period, Dr. Wells found solace and strength in her patients' unwavering support. They rallied behind her, sharing their stories of transformation and expressing gratitude for the relief they had found through her holistic approach. Their testimonials became a powerful weapon against the skeptics, serving as living proof of the efficacy of her methods.

Moreover, Dr. Wells' dedication and resilience inspired others within the medical community. Some open-minded practitioners, intrigued by her success, began to explore integrative approaches themselves. They recognized the limitations of conventional treatments and sought to bridge the gap between traditional and alternative medicine.

As the storm raged on, Dr. Wells remained steadfast, weathering each challenge with grace and determination. She understood that true progress often comes at a cost, and she was willing to pay the price to pave the way for a more holistic and compassionate approach to healthcare.

Through it all, her unwavering belief in the healing power of nature and her commitment to her patients' well-being remained her guiding light. She refused to be deterred by the resistance, knowing that every obstacle she overcame brought her one step closer to a paradigm shift in the way hypothyroidism, and perhaps even other chronic conditions, were treated.

9.4 Unwavering Determination

As the scrutiny from the medical establishment intensified, Dr. Sarah Wells found herself at a crossroads. The path she had chosen, one of holistic healing and natural remedies, was met with skepticism and resistance from those who clung to conventional methods. Yet, her unwavering determination to provide her patients with the best possible care fueled her resolve to continue forging ahead.

The challenges she faced were not merely external; they were also internal battles of self-doubt and uncertainty. In the quiet moments, when the weight of opposition seemed overwhelming, Dr. Wells would remind herself of the profound transformations she had witnessed in her patients. The renewed vitality, the shedding of excess weight, the restoration of emotional equilibrium – these were not mere anecdotes but tangible evidence of the power of nature's healing embrace.

With each patient's success story, her conviction grew stronger. She knew that she was not merely challenging the status quo; she was pioneering a new era of integrative healthcare, one that acknowledged the intricate interplay between mind, body, and spirit. It was a path that demanded courage, resilience, and an unwavering belief in the wisdom of nature.

Dr. Wells found solace in the words of ancient healers who had walked this path before her. Their teachings, once dismissed as antiquated, now resonated with a profound truth. She realized that she was not alone in her quest; she was part of a lineage of visionaries who had dared to challenge the boundaries of conventional wisdom.

As she delved deeper into the teachings of these ancient sages, she discovered a wealth of knowledge that had been overlooked or forgotten by modern medicine. Herbs that had been used for centuries to support thyroid function, dietary practices that promoted hormonal balance, and mind-body techniques that harnessed the body's innate healing capabilities – these were the tools that Dr. Wells wielded with precision and care.

Yet, even as she embraced these time-honored traditions, she remained open to the insights of modern science. She understood that true healing required a harmonious integration of ancient wisdom and contemporary knowledge. It was this holistic approach that set her apart from those who clung to rigid dogmas, whether conventional or alternative.

With each patient who walked through the doors of her clinic, Dr. Wells renewed her commitment to their well-being. She listened intently to their stories, their struggles, and their hopes. In their eyes, she saw not just physical ailments but the profound impact that hypothyroidism had on their lives – the emotional turmoil, the sense of isolation, and the loss of vitality.

It was this deep empathy that fueled her determination to find solutions that went beyond merely managing symptoms. She sought to address the root causes of imbalance, to restore harmony within the body, and to empower her patients to reclaim their health and their lives.

As the challenges mounted, Dr. Wells found strength in the unwavering support of her colleagues and the growing community of like-minded individuals who believed in the power of holistic healing. Together, they formed a united front, a beacon of hope for those seeking alternatives to the conventional approach.

In the face of skepticism and scrutiny, Dr. Wells remained steadfast in her convictions. She knew that the path she had chosen was not an easy one, but it was a path worth walking. With each step, she paved the way for a future where integrative healthcare was not merely an alternative but an integral part of the healing journey.

Her unwavering determination was not born of stubbornness or defiance; it was a testament to her deep belief in the transformative power of nature and her commitment to the well-being of her patients. In a world that often prioritized expediency over true healing, Dr. Wells stood as a beacon of hope, guiding others towards a more holistic and compassionate approach to healthcare.

9.5 Forging Ahead

As the scrutiny from the medical establishment intensified, Dr. Sarah Wells found herself at a crossroads. The path she had chosen, though paved with the purest intentions, was riddled with obstacles and resistance. Yet, her unwavering determination to provide holistic healing for those suffering from hypothyroidism burned brighter than ever before.

The opposition she faced was not merely a clash of ideologies but a battle against deeply entrenched beliefs and systems. The conventional medical community, with its reliance on synthetic medications and standardized protocols, viewed her integrative approach as a threat to their established norms. They questioned the validity of her methods, demanding rigorous scientific proof that nature's remedies could effectively treat a condition as complex as hypothyroidism.

Dr. Wells understood the weight of their skepticism. After all, she had once been a part of the very system she now challenged. However, her experiences with patients and her exploration of ancient healing traditions had opened her eyes to a world of possibilities that conventional medicine had long overlooked.

With each patient who found relief through her holistic treatments, Dr. Wells's conviction grew stronger. She witnessed firsthand the transformative power of dietary changes, herbal supplements, acupuncture, and stress-reduction techniques. The testimonies of those who had regained their vitality, shed excess weight, and reclaimed emotional equilibrium were living proof that her approach held merit.

Yet, the path forward was fraught with challenges. Navigating the bureaucratic maze of regulations and guidelines was a daunting task. Securing funding for research and clinical trials was an uphill battle, as many institutions were reluctant to invest in unconventional methods. Even within her own clinic, there were whispers of doubt and skepticism from those who clung to traditional practices.

Despite these obstacles, Dr. Wells remained steadfast in her mission. She understood that true progress often came at the cost of resistance and adversity. Her unwavering determination was fueled by the belief that every individual deserved access to holistic healing, free from the constraints of a one-size-fits-all approach.

With each step forward, Dr. Wells forged ahead, undeterred by the naysayers and critics. She sought allies in unexpected places, forming collaborations with like-minded practitioners and researchers who shared her vision. Together, they embarked on a journey to bridge the divide between conventional and alternative medicine, paving the way for a new era of integrative healthcare.

Dr. Wells's clinic became a beacon of hope for those seeking a more comprehensive approach to thyroid health. She meticulously documented each patient's journey, gathering data and evidence to support her methods. Every success story added to the growing body of knowledge, strengthening her resolve and inspiring others to embrace the power of holistic healing.

As the demand for her services grew, Dr. Wells expanded her reach, offering workshops and seminars to educate both patients and healthcare professionals alike. She shared her insights and experiences, challenging long-held beliefs and encouraging open-mindedness towards alternative therapies.

Through her unwavering perseverance, Dr. Wells not only forged a path for herself but also paved the way for a paradigm shift in the treatment of hypothyroidism. Her courage and conviction inspired others to question the status quo and seek out integrative solutions that addressed the root causes of imbalance, rather than merely masking symptoms.

In the face of adversity, Dr. Sarah Wells stood tall, her vision unwavering, her determination unbreakable. She understood that true healing extended beyond the confines of a single approach, embracing the wisdom of nature and the inherent resilience of the human spirit. With each step forward, she forged a legacy of hope, empowering others to embark on their own journeys towards holistic wellness.

Chapter 10: Allies in the Fray

10.1 Unexpected Support

In the midst of the mounting resistance against her unconventional approach, Dr. Sarah Wells found herself unexpectedly bolstered by a wave of support from an unlikely source. As the news of her holistic clinic and its remarkable success stories spread, a growing number of patients began to seek her out, drawn by the promise of a natural and integrative approach to thyroid health.

Among these new allies was a group of individuals who had long been disillusioned with the limitations of conventional medicine. They were a diverse collective, united by their shared experiences of frustration, misdiagnosis, and the debilitating effects of hypothyroidism on their lives.

One such ally was Emily, a young woman in her late twenties who had been struggling with thyroid issues since her teenage years. Despite a barrage of tests and medications, her symptoms persisted, leaving her exhausted, depressed, and unable to fully embrace the vibrant life she had once envisioned.

"I had almost given up hope," Emily confessed, her eyes brimming with tears. "I felt like a prisoner in my own body, and no one seemed to understand the depth of my suffering."

It was through a chance encounter with one of Dr. Wells's former patients that Emily learned of the holistic approach to thyroid care. Intrigued by the prospect of a natural solution, she made an appointment at the clinic, her heart filled with cautious optimism.

As Emily recounted her journey during her initial consultation, Dr. Wells listened intently, her empathy and understanding evident in her warm gaze. Together, they crafted a personalized treatment plan that encompassed dietary modifications, herbal supplements, and mindfulness practices.

"For the first time in years, I felt truly heard and understood," Emily shared, her voice tinged with gratitude. "Dr. Wells not only addressed my physical symptoms but also acknowledged the emotional toll this condition had taken on me."

Emily's story was just one of many that began to resonate within the community, sparking a groundswell of interest in Dr. Wells's pioneering work. Word spread rapidly through social media platforms, support groups, and personal networks, as individuals sought solace and hope in the face of their ongoing struggles.

Among the unexpected allies were also healthcare professionals who had grown disenchanted with the limitations of conventional medicine. These individuals, ranging from nurses to alternative therapists, were drawn to Dr. Wells's integrative approach and the profound impact it had on her patients' lives.

One such ally was Dr. Marcus Daniels, a respected acupuncturist with decades of experience in the field of holistic healing. Initially skeptical of Dr. Wells's methods, he found himself captivated by the depth of her knowledge and the remarkable results she achieved.

"I have witnessed firsthand the transformative power of integrative medicine," Dr. Daniels remarked, his voice resonating with conviction. "Dr. Wells's work is a testament to the healing potential that lies within nature and the human body's innate ability to heal itself when given the proper support."

As the ranks of allies swelled, a sense of community began to take root around Dr. Wells's clinic. Support groups formed, allowing patients to share their experiences, offer encouragement, and celebrate their collective victories over the challenges posed by hypothyroidism.

10.2 Strength in Numbers

As Dr. Sarah Wells navigated the turbulent waters of opposition and skepticism, she found solace in the knowledge that she was not alone in her quest for holistic healing. Gradually, a network of like-minded individuals emerged, united by their shared belief in the power of natural remedies and their unwavering commitment to challenging the status quo.

One such ally was Dr. Emily Hawthorne, a renowned herbalist and naturopathic physician from the Pacific Northwest. With decades of experience in the field, Dr. Hawthorne had witnessed firsthand the transformative effects of plant-based medicines on her patients' well-being. Her expertise in formulating herbal blends and tinctures proved invaluable to Dr. Wells's practice, providing a wealth of knowledge that complemented her own research.

Their collaboration blossomed into a deep friendship, fueled by their shared passion for holistic healing and their determination to offer patients a comprehensive approach to thyroid disorders. Together, they organized workshops and seminars, educating both healthcare professionals and the public about the benefits of integrating natural remedies into conventional treatment plans.

Another ally emerged in the form of Dr. Amir Khan, a respected acupuncturist from the heart of New York City. With his extensive training in Traditional Chinese Medicine, Dr. Khan brought a unique perspective to the team, offering insights into the delicate balance of energy and its impact on thyroid function. His gentle yet effective acupuncture treatments became an integral part of the clinic's holistic approach, helping patients achieve a greater sense of harmony and well-being.

As word of their innovative methods spread, more healthcare professionals joined the ranks, each bringing their own unique expertise and passion to the table. Dr. Samantha Rodriguez, a yoga instructor and mindfulness coach, introduced patients to the healing power of breathwork and meditation, teaching them techniques to manage stress and cultivate inner peace – essential components for thyroid health.

Together, this diverse group of practitioners formed a formidable force, their collective knowledge and experience creating a comprehensive approach to thyroid care that addressed not only the physical symptoms but also the emotional and spiritual aspects of the condition.

The strength of their alliance was evident in the countless success stories that emerged from the clinic. Patients who had previously struggled with debilitating fatigue, weight fluctuations, and emotional turmoil found newfound vitality and balance through the integrative treatments offered by this dedicated team.

One such patient, Emily Thompson, had spent years bouncing from doctor to doctor, desperately seeking relief from her hypothyroidism. After countless rounds of synthetic medications and frustrating side effects, she found her way to Dr. Wells's clinic. Through a combination of dietary changes, herbal supplements, and acupuncture treatments, Emily's life was transformed. Her energy levels soared, her weight stabilized, and her mood improved dramatically.

"I had almost given up hope," Emily shared, her eyes brimming with tears of gratitude. "But this team of incredible healers showed me that there was another way – a path back to wellness that honored my body and my spirit. I am forever grateful for their dedication and their unwavering belief in the power of natural healing."

Stories like Emily's served as a powerful testament to the efficacy of the holistic approach championed by Dr. Wells and her allies. Each patient's journey was a triumph over adversity, a reminder that when conventional methods fall short, the wisdom of nature and the strength of a united front can pave the way for true healing.

As their collective voice grew louder, the resistance they faced began to wane. Slowly but surely, the medical establishment took notice, and a shift in perspective began to emerge. The once-unconventional methods they advocated were now being recognized as valuable complements to traditional treatments, offering patients a more comprehensive and personalized approach to their care.

In the face of adversity, Dr. Wells and her allies had forged an unbreakable bond, a testament to the power of collaboration and the unwavering pursuit of healing. Their strength in numbers had not only transformed countless lives but had also paved the way for a new era of integrative healthcare, where the boundaries between conventional and alternative medicine blurred, and the well-being of the patient remained the ultimate priority.

10.3 Uniting Voices

As Dr. Sarah Wells navigated the challenges of establishing her holistic approach to thyroid care, she found herself increasingly emboldened by the growing support from unexpected allies. What had once felt like a solitary journey was now transforming into a collective movement, fueled by the shared experiences and unwavering determination of those who had witnessed the transformative power of natural healing.

Among her newfound allies were patients who had experienced remarkable improvements in their health and well-being. Their stories resonated deeply, serving as living testaments to the efficacy of Dr. Wells's integrative methods. These individuals became passionate advocates, sharing their journeys with others and igniting a spark of hope in those who had long struggled with the debilitating effects of hypothyroidism.

One such ally was Emily, a young woman whose life had been consumed by fatigue, brain fog, and unexplained weight gain. After years of frustration with conventional treatments, she had stumbled upon Dr. Wells's clinic, initially skeptical but willing to try anything that offered a glimmer of hope. Within months of embracing the holistic approach, Emily's energy levels soared, her mental clarity returned, and her once-stubborn weight began to shed effortlessly.

"It was like emerging from a fog that had enveloped my life for years," Emily recalled. "Dr. Wells's approach not only addressed my physical symptoms but also helped me regain control over my emotional well-being. I felt truly alive again."

Emily's story resonated with countless others who had endured similar struggles. Her unwavering gratitude and advocacy for Dr. Wells's work inspired others to seek out the clinic, creating a ripple effect that amplified the movement's reach.

Another unexpected ally emerged in the form of Dr. Marcus Daniels, a respected endocrinologist who had initially been skeptical of Dr. Wells's unconventional methods. However, after witnessing the remarkable transformations in several of his patients who had sought integrative care, Dr. Daniels found himself intrigued and open to exploring alternative approaches.

"As a physician, my primary responsibility is to alleviate suffering and promote healing," Dr. Daniels explained. "While I was initially hesitant about Dr. Wells's methods, the results spoke for themselves. I couldn't ignore the profound improvements my patients were experiencing."

Dr. Daniels became a valuable ally, lending his expertise and credibility to the movement. His willingness to engage in open dialogue and collaborate with Dr. Wells helped bridge the gap between conventional and holistic medicine, paving the way for a more inclusive and integrative approach to thyroid care.

As the movement gained momentum, other healthcare professionals, researchers, and advocates began to take notice. Naturopaths, herbalists, and holistic practitioners from around the world rallied behind Dr. Wells's work, sharing their own insights and experiences. Collectively, they formed a powerful network, united by a common goal: to revolutionize the way hypothyroidism and other thyroid disorders were understood and treated.

This diverse coalition of voices amplified the message of holistic healing, reaching far beyond the confines of Dr. Wells's clinic. Through conferences, seminars, and online platforms, they shared their knowledge and experiences, empowering individuals to take control of their health and explore the vast potential of natural remedies.

The united voices resonated with those who had felt dismissed or marginalized by the conventional medical system. Patients who had struggled for years with unresolved symptoms found solace and validation in the stories shared by this growing community. They were no longer alone in their journey, but part of a movement that celebrated the body's innate ability to heal when provided with the right tools and support.

As the movement gained traction, it became increasingly difficult for the medical establishment to ignore the growing body of evidence and personal testimonies. The collective voices of patients, healthcare professionals, and advocates echoed with a resounding call for change, challenging the status quo and demanding a more inclusive and holistic approach to thyroid care.

In the face of adversity, Dr. Sarah Wells and her allies stood united, their voices amplifying the message of hope and healing. Together, they were paving the way for a paradigm shift in healthcare, one that embraced the wisdom of nature and the power of integrative medicine.

10.4 A Shared Vision

As Dr. Wells navigated the challenges posed by the medical establishment, she found solace in the support of like-minded individuals who shared her vision of holistic healing. Their collective voices resonated with a shared belief in the power of nature and the importance of integrating traditional and alternative approaches to healthcare.

One such ally was Dr. Amelia Nguyen, a renowned acupuncturist and herbalist from the Pacific Northwest. Dr. Nguyen had spent decades studying ancient Eastern healing practices and witnessed firsthand the transformative effects of these modalities on her patients. She was a fierce advocate for the integration of traditional Chinese medicine into mainstream healthcare.

When Dr. Wells first met Dr. Nguyen at a conference on integrative medicine, they immediately connected over their shared passion for natural healing. Dr. Nguyen was captivated by Dr. Wells's pioneering work in treating hypothyroidism through holistic means, and she recognized the immense potential for collaboration.

"Sarah, your approach to thyroid health is truly revolutionary," Dr. Nguyen exclaimed, her eyes sparkling with excitement. "I've seen countless patients struggle with the side effects of synthetic medications, and your emphasis on natural remedies and lifestyle changes could be the answer they've been seeking."

Dr. Wells was equally impressed by Dr. Nguyen's extensive knowledge and expertise. "Amelia, your mastery of acupuncture and herbal medicine is truly inspiring," she responded. "I believe that by combining our strengths, we can create a powerful synergy that will benefit countless individuals suffering from thyroid disorders."

From that moment on, Dr. Wells and Dr. Nguyen became steadfast allies, united by their shared vision of integrating traditional and modern healing modalities. They began collaborating on research projects, exploring the synergistic effects of herbal remedies and acupuncture in managing hypothyroidism.

Their partnership extended beyond the realm of research, as they co-founded a non-profit organization dedicated to promoting holistic healthcare and educating the public about the benefits of natural therapies. Together, they organized seminars, workshops, and community outreach programs, spreading their message of holistic wellness to a broader audience.

As their movement gained momentum, more healthcare professionals and advocates joined their ranks, each bringing their unique perspectives and expertise to the table. Dr. Marcus Hernandez, a naturopathic physician from the Southwest, shared his insights on the role of nutrition and dietary interventions in thyroid health. Dr. Jasmine Khan, a yoga instructor and mindfulness coach, contributed her knowledge of stress-reduction techniques and their impact on overall well-being.

The diverse backgrounds and experiences of these allies created a rich tapestry of knowledge and wisdom, weaving together ancient traditions and modern scientific advancements. Their shared vision transcended individual disciplines, fostering a collaborative environment where ideas could flourish and innovative solutions could emerge.

Together, they formed a powerful coalition, a united front against the resistance they faced from the conventional medical establishment. Their collective voices amplified the call for a more inclusive and integrative approach to healthcare, one that embraced the healing power of nature while respecting the advancements of modern medicine.

As they stood side by side, their shared vision became a beacon of hope for countless individuals seeking alternative paths to wellness. Their unwavering commitment to holistic healing inspired others to question the status quo and explore the vast potential of natural remedies.

Through their collaborative efforts, Dr. Wells and her allies were not only transforming the landscape of thyroid care but also paving the way for a broader paradigm shift in healthcare. They embodied the spirit of innovation and compassion, reminding the world that true healing often lies in the harmonious integration of diverse perspectives and approaches.

10.5 Empowering Others

As Dr. Wells navigated the challenges posed by the medical establishment, she realized that the true strength of her mission lay in empowering others to embrace holistic wellness. Her journey had taught her that healing was not a solitary endeavor but a collective effort, fueled by the shared experiences and insights of those who had walked a similar path.

In the cozy confines of her clinic, Dr. Wells gathered a diverse group of individuals who had been touched by the transformative power of natural remedies. Some were former patients, now thriving and eager to share their stories of recovery. Others were practitioners of alternative medicine, each bringing their unique perspectives and expertise to the table.

The atmosphere was electric, filled with a palpable sense of camaraderie and purpose. Dr. Wells welcomed them all with open arms, her eyes alight with the fire of determination that had carried her through the most daunting of obstacles.

"My friends," she began, her voice resonating with conviction, "we stand at a crossroads. The path we have chosen is not an easy one, but it is a path of truth, of healing, and of hope."

She paused, allowing her words to sink in, before continuing, "For too long, we have been silenced by those who refuse to acknowledge the wisdom of nature's bounty. But today, we rise together, united in our belief that there is a better way – a way that honors the intricate balance of mind, body, and spirit."

A murmur of agreement rippled through the room, as each person nodded in solidarity, their eyes shining with a newfound sense of purpose.

"We are not alone in this fight," Dr. Wells declared. "There are countless others out there, yearning for a holistic approach to wellness, seeking solace in the embrace of nature's remedies. It is our duty, our calling, to be their beacons of hope, to guide them towards a path of true healing."

With a wave of her hand, she invited the group to share their stories, their triumphs, and their struggles. One by one, they stepped forward, their voices weaving a tapestry of resilience and transformation.

Emily, a young woman who had once been crippled by the debilitating effects of hypothyroidism, spoke of how Dr. Wells's integrative approach had not only alleviated her physical symptoms but had also rekindled her zest for life. "I was a mere shadow of myself," she confessed, "until Dr. Wells showed me the power of nature's healing touch."

Jacob, an acupuncturist with decades of experience, shared his insights into the ancient art of balancing the body's energy flow. "Western medicine has its place," he acknowledged, "but it cannot heal what it does not understand – the intricate web of energy that binds us to the natural world."

As each person spoke, a sense of unity grew stronger, a collective understanding that their individual journeys were part of a greater movement, a revolution in healthcare that promised to reshape the way we perceive and treat illness.

Dr. Wells listened intently, her heart swelling with pride and determination. These were not just allies in her fight; they were warriors, each armed with their own unique experiences and knowledge, ready to take up the mantle of holistic healing.

"Together, we will blaze a trail," she declared, her voice ringing with conviction. "We will educate, inspire, and empower others to embrace the healing power of nature. We will challenge the status quo, not with aggression, but with compassion and understanding."

She looked around the room, meeting the gaze of each individual, her eyes shining with a fierce determination. "This is not just a battle for our own well-being; it is a fight for the future of healthcare, for the generations to come. We must be the change we wish to see in the world, and together, we will leave an indelible mark on the path to true wellness."

As the gathering drew to a close, a sense of unity and purpose lingered in the air. Each person left with a renewed sense of determination, empowered by the knowledge that they were part of something greater – a movement that would reshape the landscape of healthcare, one step, one life at a time.

In that moment, Dr. Wells knew that her journey had transcended the confines of her clinic. She had ignited a spark, a flame that would burn brightly, illuminating the way for countless others seeking solace in the embrace of nature's healing touch.

Chapter 11: A Paradigm Shift

11.1 Changing Perspectives

As the sun rose over the bustling city of Metropolis, a new dawn was breaking in the realm of healthcare. Dr. Sarah Wells's unwavering dedication to holistic wellness had sparked a profound shift in perspectives, one that would forever change the way thyroid disorders were approached and treated.

For years, the medical establishment had clung to a narrow view of hypothyroidism, relying solely on synthetic medications and dismissing the potential of natural remedies. However, the remarkable results achieved by Dr. Wells's integrative approach could no longer be ignored. Patients who had once struggled with debilitating symptoms were now thriving, their lives transformed by the power of nature's healing touch.

Word of Dr. Wells's success spread like wildfire, igniting a flame of curiosity and hope within the medical community. Physicians who had once been skeptical began to open their minds, intrigued by the possibility of a more comprehensive approach to thyroid health. They witnessed firsthand the profound impact of dietary changes, herbal supplements, and stress-reduction techniques on their patients' well-being.

As the demand for integrative care grew, a ripple effect began to take hold. Medical schools and research institutions started to recognize the value of incorporating holistic practices into their curricula and studies. Conferences and seminars were organized, bringing together experts from diverse fields to share their knowledge and experiences.

The shift in perspective was not limited to the medical realm alone. Patients, too, began to embrace a more holistic view of their health. They sought out practitioners who could provide personalized, comprehensive care that addressed not just their physical symptoms but also their emotional and spiritual well-being.

Slowly but surely, the once-rigid boundaries between conventional and alternative medicine began to blur. Physicians and naturopaths found common ground, recognizing that true healing often required a multifaceted approach that combined the best of both worlds.

Dr. Wells's clinic became a beacon of hope, attracting patients from far and wide who yearned for a more compassionate and integrative approach to their care. Her dedicated team of practitioners worked tirelessly, tailoring treatments to each individual's unique needs and circumstances.

The transformation extended beyond the clinic's walls, as Dr. Wells and her colleagues became advocates for a paradigm shift in healthcare. They spoke at conferences, authored research papers, and engaged in public outreach efforts, spreading the message of holistic wellness and the importance of addressing the root causes of illness, not just treating symptoms.

As the movement gained momentum, a new era of healthcare began to take shape – one that embraced the wisdom of ancient healing traditions while harnessing the power of modern science. Patients were empowered to take an active role in their own healing journeys, supported by a collaborative team of practitioners who recognized the intricate connections between mind, body, and spirit.

The road to this paradigm shift was not without its challenges, but Dr. Wells's unwavering determination and the growing body of evidence supporting her approach paved the way for lasting change. Each patient who experienced the transformative power of holistic wellness became a living testament to the efficacy of this integrative approach, inspiring others to embrace a more comprehensive view of health and healing.

11.2 Embracing Integration

As Dr. Wells's holistic approach to treating hypothyroidism gained traction, a profound shift began to take shape within the medical community. The once-rigid boundaries between conventional and alternative medicine started to blur, paving the way for a more integrative and inclusive approach to healthcare.

At first, the resistance was palpable. Skeptics questioned the validity of Dr. Wells's methods, citing a lack of scientific evidence and adherence to traditional protocols. However, the transformative results witnessed by her patients could not be ignored. One by one, open-minded healthcare professionals began to take notice, their curiosity piqued by the remarkable improvements in their patients' overall well-being.

Dr. Marcus Ellison, a respected endocrinologist, was among the first to embrace the potential of integrative medicine. Initially skeptical, he found himself intrigued by the holistic approach after witnessing the remarkable recovery of one of his long-term patients, who had struggled with hypothyroidism for years.

"I have to admit, when Sarah first approached me about her methods, I was hesitant," Dr. Ellison confessed. "But after seeing the profound impact it had on Mrs. Thompson, I couldn't ignore the possibility that there might be something more to explore."

Driven by a genuine desire to provide the best possible care for his patients, Dr. Ellison began collaborating with Dr. Wells, seeking to understand the intricacies of her integrative approach. Together, they embarked on a journey of knowledge-sharing, combining the strengths of conventional medicine with the wisdom of holistic healing practices.

As their partnership blossomed, they witnessed remarkable transformations in their patients' lives. The combination of dietary adjustments, herbal supplements, and stress-reduction techniques not only alleviated the symptoms of hypothyroidism but also addressed the underlying imbalances that had previously gone unnoticed.

"It was like unlocking a missing piece of the puzzle," Dr. Ellison marveled. "By addressing the whole person, not just the condition, we were able to achieve results that surpassed our expectations."

Word of their success spread rapidly, inspiring other healthcare professionals to explore the potential of integrative medicine. Slowly but surely, a shift in mindset began to take hold, as more practitioners recognized the value of a holistic approach in treating chronic conditions like hypothyroidism.

Dr. Wells's clinic became a hub of learning and collaboration, attracting physicians, nurses, and therapists from various disciplines. Together, they formed a dynamic community dedicated to advancing the field of integrative medicine, sharing insights, and developing comprehensive treatment protocols.

"It's not about abandoning conventional medicine," Dr. Wells explained. "It's about embracing the best of both worlds – utilizing the scientific rigor of modern medicine while harnessing the healing power of nature and ancient wisdom."

The integration of holistic practices into mainstream healthcare brought about a newfound sense of empowerment for patients. They were no longer passive recipients of treatment but active participants in their healing journeys. By incorporating lifestyle changes, mindfulness practices, and natural remedies, they regained control over their well-being, becoming partners in their own recovery.

As the integrative approach gained momentum, it inspired a broader cultural shift towards preventive care and holistic living. Patients began to embrace the concept of whole-body wellness, recognizing the interconnectedness of physical, emotional, and spiritual health.

"It's not just about treating a condition," one patient shared. "It's about cultivating a lifestyle that nurtures and supports our overall well-being. Dr. Wells has shown us that true healing goes beyond just managing symptoms – it's about finding balance and harmony within ourselves."

The paradigm shift toward integrative medicine was not without its challenges, but the transformative results spoke for themselves. As more healthcare professionals witnessed the positive impact on their patients' lives, the resistance gradually gave way to curiosity and a willingness to explore new avenues of healing.

In the end, Dr. Wells's pioneering work paved the way for a more compassionate and holistic approach to healthcare, one that acknowledged the complexity of the human experience and embraced the healing power of nature in harmony with modern medical advancements.

11.3 Bridging the Divide

As Dr. Wells's holistic approach to treating hypothyroidism gained traction, a remarkable shift began to unfold within the medical community. The once-rigid boundaries between conventional and alternative medicine started to blur, paving the way for a new era of integrative healthcare.

The success stories of her patients, coupled with the growing body of research supporting natural remedies, caught the attention of open-minded medical professionals. Curiosity and a genuine desire to explore new avenues for healing prompted many to seek out Dr. Wells, eager to learn from her pioneering work.

One such individual was Dr. Michael Dawson, a respected endocrinologist who had dedicated his career to the study of thyroid disorders. Initially skeptical of Dr. Wells's methods, he found himself captivated by the remarkable transformations he witnessed in her patients. Their renewed energy, weight loss, and overall improvement in quality of life challenged his long-held beliefs about the limitations of conventional treatments.

Driven by a thirst for knowledge, Dr. Dawson reached out to Dr. Wells, initiating a dialogue that would bridge the gap between their seemingly disparate worlds. Their initial conversations were laced with caution and skepticism, but as they delved deeper into the science behind natural remedies, a mutual respect began to emerge.

Dr. Wells meticulously explained the intricate mechanisms by which herbs, dietary changes, and lifestyle modifications could support thyroid function and alleviate symptoms. She shared her extensive research, citing ancient texts and modern studies that validated the efficacy of her approach. Dr. Dawson, in turn, offered his expertise in endocrinology, providing valuable insights into the complex interplay between the thyroid and the body's various systems.

As their discussions progressed, a remarkable synergy took shape. Dr. Dawson began to recognize the limitations of relying solely on synthetic medications and acknowledged the potential benefits of incorporating natural therapies into his practice. Conversely, Dr. Wells gained a deeper appreciation for the role of conventional medicine, realizing that a truly holistic approach required the integration of both worlds.

Their collaboration sparked a wave of curiosity among their colleagues, who witnessed the transformative power of this newfound partnership. Physicians from various specialties sought out Dr. Wells and Dr. Dawson, eager to learn about their integrative approach and its potential applications in their respective fields.

Conferences and seminars were organized, where Dr. Wells and Dr. Dawson shared their insights and experiences, challenging long-held beliefs and inspiring others to explore the possibilities of integrative medicine. Their presentations were met with a mix of enthusiasm and skepticism, but the seeds of change had been planted.

As more medical professionals embraced the concept of integrative care, a shift in the healthcare landscape began to take shape. Hospitals and clinics started to incorporate naturopathic practitioners, acupuncturists, and herbalists into their teams, recognizing the value of a multidisciplinary approach to patient care.

The divide between conventional and alternative medicine slowly dissolved, replaced by a collaborative spirit that prioritized the well-being of patients above all else. Doctors and practitioners from various backgrounds worked together, combining their expertise to develop personalized treatment plans that addressed the root causes of illness, rather than merely treating symptoms.

This paradigm shift extended beyond the medical realm, influencing policymakers and insurance providers to recognize the importance of integrative care. Gradually, coverage for alternative therapies became more accessible, allowing patients to explore a broader range of treatment options without financial constraints.

As the integration of conventional and alternative medicine gained momentum, a new era of healthcare emerged – one that embraced the wisdom of ancient healing traditions while harnessing the power of modern science. Dr. Wells's pioneering work had not only transformed the lives of her patients but had also catalyzed a profound shift in the way society approached health and wellness.

11.4 A New Era Dawns

As the sun rose over Metropolis, a new era dawned, one that promised to reshape the landscape of healthcare forever. Dr. Sarah Wells had embarked on a journey that challenged the very foundations of conventional medicine, and her unwavering determination had paved the way for a paradigm shift.

The air was thick with anticipation as patients, practitioners, and advocates alike gathered at the newly established Integrative Health Center. This state-of-the-art facility stood as a beacon of hope, a testament to the power of collaboration and the relentless pursuit of holistic wellness.

Dr. Wells stepped onto the podium, her eyes shining with a mixture of pride and humility. She surveyed the diverse crowd before her, each face a reminder of the countless lives touched by her work. With a deep breath, she began to speak.

"Today, we stand at the precipice of a new era in healthcare," she declared, her voice resonating with conviction. "For too long, the conventional medical system has overlooked the inherent wisdom of nature and the profound interconnectedness of mind, body, and spirit."

A hush fell over the audience as they hung onto her every word, captivated by the passion that fueled her mission.

"Through our collective efforts, we have challenged the status quo and opened the doors to a more comprehensive approach to healing," Dr. Wells continued. "No longer will we settle for treating symptoms alone; instead, we will embrace the intricate tapestry of human health, weaving together the best of modern science and ancient wisdom."

Her words struck a chord with those in attendance, resonating with their own experiences and struggles. For many, the journey to this moment had been long and arduous, filled with frustration and despair as they navigated the limitations of traditional medicine.

"The Integrative Health Center stands as a testament to our unwavering belief in the power of holistic healing," Dr. Wells declared, her voice rising with conviction. "Here, we will merge the knowledge of naturopaths, herbalists, acupuncturists, and traditional healers, creating a synergy that transcends the boundaries of any single discipline."

The audience erupted in applause, their enthusiasm a tangible force that filled the room. They had witnessed firsthand the transformative effects of Dr. Wells's approach, and now, they were part of something greater – a movement that promised to reshape the very fabric of healthcare.

"This is not merely a building; it is a sanctuary where individuals can embark on a journey of self-discovery and healing," Dr. Wells continued, her eyes shining with determination. "Within these walls, we will nurture the mind, nourish the body, and uplift the spirit, empowering each person to reclaim their vitality and embrace a life of wholeness."

As she spoke, the air crackled with energy, a palpable sense of possibility that transcended the boundaries of the physical space. This was more than just a medical facility; it was a beacon of hope, a place where the impossible became attainable, and the boundaries of healing were pushed ever further.

"Today, we stand united, a diverse tapestry of individuals woven together by a shared vision of compassionate, integrative care," Dr. Wells proclaimed, her voice resonating with conviction. "Together, we will forge a new path, one that honors the wisdom of the ages while embracing the cutting edge of modern science."

The audience rose to their feet, their thunderous applause a resounding affirmation of the journey they had embarked upon. In that moment, the Integrative Health Center became a symbol of transformation, a living embodiment of the paradigm shift that was sweeping across the healthcare landscape.

As Dr. Wells stepped down from the podium, she was greeted by a sea of smiling faces, each one a testament to the power of perseverance and the indomitable spirit of those who dared to challenge convention. This was not the end of a journey, but the beginning of a new era – an era where healing transcended boundaries, and the pursuit of holistic wellness became a beacon of hope for generations to come.

11.5 Celebrating Triumph

The air was electric with anticipation as Dr. Wells stood before a packed auditorium, her heart swelling with pride. The journey that had once seemed like an uphill battle against the establishment had now blossomed into a movement, a paradigm shift that was reshaping the landscape of thyroid care.

As she scanned the sea of faces before her, she saw a tapestry of individuals united by a common goal – to embrace a holistic approach to wellness. Physicians, researchers, patients, and advocates from around the globe had gathered to celebrate the triumphs of integrative medicine and its impact on thyroid disorders.

Dr. Wells took a deep breath, her mind awash with memories of the challenges she had faced, the skepticism she had endured, and the unwavering determination that had fueled her every step. It was a moment to reflect on the countless lives that had been transformed by the power of natural healing.

"Friends, colleagues, and fellow seekers of truth," she began, her voice resonating with conviction. "Today, we stand at the precipice of a new era in healthcare, one where the boundaries between conventional and alternative medicine are blurred, and the focus is on the individual's journey to wholeness."

A wave of applause rippled through the auditorium, echoing the shared sentiment of those present. Dr. Wells allowed the energy to wash over her, drawing strength from the collective spirit of the gathering.

"When I first embarked on this path, I was met with skepticism and resistance," she continued. "The medical establishment viewed my methods as unconventional, unproven, and even dangerous. But I refused to be deterred, for I had witnessed firsthand the transformative power of nature's remedies."

She paused, her gaze sweeping across the rapt audience, many of whom nodded in recognition of their own struggles against the status quo.

"It was a journey paved with challenges, but every obstacle only strengthened my resolve. Each patient who found relief through our integrative approach became a beacon of hope, a testament to the efficacy of holistic healing."

Dr. Wells gestured towards the stage, where a group of individuals stood, each a living embodiment of the triumph over thyroid disorders. Their faces radiated with vitality, their eyes shining with gratitude.

"These remarkable individuals are living proof of what can be achieved when we embrace the synergy between conventional and natural medicine," she declared. "Their stories are a tapestry woven with resilience, perseverance, and the unwavering belief that there is always a path to wellness."

As the crowd erupted in thunderous applause, Dr. Wells felt a surge of emotion, her heart overflowing with gratitude for the allies who had stood by her side, the patients who had placed their trust in her, and the countless individuals who had contributed to this paradigm shift.

"Today, we celebrate not just our victories, but the courage it took to challenge the status quo," she said, her voice ringing with conviction. "We celebrate the power of collaboration, the strength of diversity, and the unwavering commitment to putting the well-being of our patients above all else."

The auditorium echoed with cheers and applause, a collective affirmation of the shared values that had brought them together. Dr. Wells allowed the energy to wash over her, basking in the warmth of a community that had once seemed like a distant dream.

"Let this moment be a testament to the resilience of the human spirit," she declared, her eyes shining with determination. "Let it serve as a reminder that when we open our minds to new possibilities and embrace the wisdom of nature, we can unlock the true potential of healing."

As the applause thundered on, Dr. Wells felt a profound sense of gratitude for the journey that had led her to this moment. It was a triumph not just for herself, but for every individual who had dared to challenge the status quo, to seek out alternative paths to wellness, and to embrace the healing power of nature.

In that moment, she knew that the paradigm shift was not just a fleeting trend, but a movement that would continue to gain momentum, reshaping the landscape of healthcare and ushering in a new era of integrative medicine. It was a triumph not just for the present, but for generations to come, a legacy of hope and healing that would continue to inspire and empower those who dared to dream of a world where holistic wellness was the norm, not the exception.

Chapter 12: A Legacy of Hope

12.1 Inspiring Future Generations

As Dr. Sarah Wells stood in the midst of her thriving clinic, she couldn't help but reflect on the incredible journey that had led her to this moment. What had once been a seed of doubt in the conventional approach to treating hypothyroidism had blossomed into a flourishing practice, dedicated to holistic wellness and the power of natural healing.

The walls of the clinic were adorned with testimonials from patients whose lives had been transformed by Dr. Wells's pioneering methods. Each story was a testament to the resilience of the human spirit and the body's innate ability to heal when given the right tools and guidance.

But for Dr. Wells, the true legacy of her work extended far beyond the confines of her clinic. She had embarked on a mission to inspire future generations of healthcare professionals to embrace a more integrative and compassionate approach to medicine.

Through her writings, lectures, and mentorship programs, Dr. Wells shared her knowledge and experiences with aspiring naturopaths, physicians, and holistic practitioners. She encouraged them to challenge the status quo, to question the limitations of conventional medicine, and to explore the vast potential of natural remedies.

"The medical field is ever-evolving," she would often say, "and it is our responsibility to remain open-minded and adaptable, always seeking new ways to alleviate suffering and promote true wellness."

Dr. Wells's teachings resonated deeply with those who felt disillusioned by the limitations of the current healthcare system. Her words ignited a fire within them, fueling their determination to forge a new path and embrace a more holistic approach to healing.

One such student, Emily, had initially pursued a career in conventional medicine, but found herself disillusioned by the overreliance on pharmaceuticals and the lack of focus on preventative care. Inspired by

Dr. Wells's teachings, Emily decided to switch gears and pursue a degree in naturopathic medicine.

"Dr. Wells opened my eyes to the incredible power of nature's remedies," Emily shared. "She taught me that true healing goes beyond simply treating symptoms; it involves addressing the root causes of imbalance and empowering individuals to take an active role in their own well-being."

Another student, Marcus, had struggled with chronic health issues for years, bouncing from one specialist to another without finding lasting relief. It wasn't until he encountered Dr. Wells's work that he discovered the transformative potential of integrative medicine.

"Dr. Wells's approach resonated with me on a profound level," Marcus explained. "She showed me that healing is a journey, and that by embracing a holistic lifestyle and harnessing the wisdom of nature, we can achieve a state of true vitality."

As Dr. Wells's teachings spread, a ripple effect began to take shape. Her students went on to establish their own practices, clinics, and educational programs, each one carrying the torch of holistic wellness and spreading the message of hope and healing.

In the years that followed, Dr. Wells's legacy continued to grow, inspiring generations of healthcare professionals to embrace a more compassionate and integrative approach to medicine. Her unwavering dedication to empowering individuals and promoting natural healing had sparked a movement that would forever change the landscape of healthcare.

12.2 Spreading the Message

As Dr. Sarah Wells stood before the auditorium filled with eager medical students, she couldn't help but feel a sense of pride and purpose. The journey that had begun with a single seed of doubt had blossomed into a movement, inspiring countless individuals to embrace a holistic approach to wellness.

"My dear friends," she began, her voice resonating with conviction, "the path we have walked together has been one of discovery, perseverance, and ultimately, triumph. We have challenged the boundaries of conventional medicine and paved the way for a new era of integrative healthcare."

The students leaned forward, captivated by her words, their eyes shining with the same determination that had fueled Dr. Wells's own quest. She knew that these young minds represented the future of medicine, and it was her mission to equip them with the knowledge and wisdom she had gained through her pioneering work.

"When I first embarked on this journey, I was met with skepticism and resistance," she continued. "The medical establishment viewed my methods as unconventional, unproven, and even dangerous. But I refused to be deterred, for I had witnessed the transformative power of nature's healing touch."

Dr. Wells recounted the stories of her patients, each one a testament to the efficacy of holistic treatments for thyroid disorders. She spoke of the fatigue that had melted away, the emotional turmoil that had dissipated, and the radiant vitality that had been restored – all through the harmonious integration of dietary changes, herbal remedies, acupuncture, and stress-reduction techniques.

"These remarkable journeys of healing were not mere coincidences," she emphasized. "They were the result of a deep understanding of the human body's innate ability to heal itself, when provided with the right tools and nourishment."

As she looked out at the sea of faces before her, Dr. Wells saw a reflection of her own determination and passion. These students were the torchbearers of a new era, one in which conventional and alternative medicine would coexist in a harmonious dance, each complementing the other's strengths.

"The path ahead will not be easy," she cautioned. "You will encounter resistance, skepticism, and even outright opposition. But never lose sight of your purpose – to alleviate suffering and promote true wellness, in body, mind, and spirit."

Dr. Wells implored the students to embrace diversity in their approach to healing, to remain open-minded and curious, and to never stop learning. She encouraged them to seek out mentors, both in the conventional and alternative realms, and to forge their own paths, guided by compassion and a thirst for knowledge.

"Remember, my friends, that true healing is not merely the absence of disease, but the harmonious balance of all aspects of our being," she said, her voice resonating with conviction. "It is our sacred duty to guide our patients toward this state of wholeness, using every tool at our disposal, be it conventional or alternative."

As the lecture drew to a close, the auditorium erupted in thunderous applause. Dr. Wells basked in the energy of the room, knowing that her message had taken root in the hearts and minds of these future healers. They would carry the torch of holistic wellness, spreading its light to every corner of the world.

In the days and weeks that followed, Dr. Wells received countless messages from students, each one expressing gratitude for her wisdom and inspiration. Some shared their own stories of personal transformation, while others sought guidance on integrating holistic practices into their future careers.

With each interaction, Dr. Wells felt a renewed sense of purpose. Her legacy was not merely the clinic she had built or the patients she had treated, but the ripples of change that would continue to spread, touching the lives of countless individuals in search of true wellness.

As she looked to the future, Dr. Wells knew that her work was far from over. There were still battles to be fought, minds to be opened, and lives to be transformed. But she was no longer alone in this quest. She had ignited a fire within the hearts of a new generation of healers, and together, they would blaze a trail toward a more compassionate, integrative, and holistic approach to healthcare.

12.3 Nurturing Compassion

As the sun's golden rays filtered through the large windows of the clinic, Dr. Sarah Wells sat in her office, reflecting on the incredible journey that had led her to this point. The once-empty space had transformed into a thriving sanctuary of healing, where patients found solace and hope in the embrace of nature's wisdom.

Over the years, Dr. Wells had witnessed countless transformations, as individuals who had once been weighed down by the debilitating effects of hypothyroidism reclaimed their vitality and zest for life. Each success story fueled her determination to nurture compassion and spread the message of holistic wellness far and wide.

One such story that stood out in her mind was that of Emily, a young woman who had struggled with hypothyroidism since her teenage years. Emily had been through a rollercoaster of conventional treatments, each one leaving her with a new set of side effects and little relief. It wasn't until she stumbled upon Dr. Wells's clinic that her life began to change.

With a personalized treatment plan that incorporated dietary changes, herbal supplements, and mindfulness practices, Emily slowly but surely regained her energy and emotional balance. Dr. Wells vividly remembered the day Emily walked into her office, her eyes sparkling with newfound joy, and embraced her with tears of gratitude.

"You've given me back my life, Dr. Wells," Emily had said. "I never thought I'd feel this good again."

Moments like these reminded Dr. Wells of the profound impact her work had on people's lives. It was a responsibility she carried with utmost reverence, understanding that each patient who walked through the clinic's doors was entrusting her with their well-being.

As she looked around her office, adorned with framed certificates and accolades, Dr. Wells couldn't help but feel a sense of pride in how far she had come. However, she knew that her journey was far from over. There were still countless individuals out there who needed guidance and support on their path to holistic healing.

With a renewed sense of purpose, Dr. Wells began to envision ways to expand her reach and nurture compassion on a larger scale. She dreamed of establishing a comprehensive training program for healthcare professionals, where they could learn the principles of integrative medicine and the art of treating the whole person, not just the symptoms.

Through this program, she hoped to inspire a new generation of practitioners who would embrace a compassionate and holistic approach to healthcare. By equipping them with the knowledge and tools to address the root causes of imbalances, they could empower their patients to take an active role in their healing journey.

Dr. Wells also envisioned creating a series of educational resources, ranging from books and online courses to workshops and seminars. These resources would not only cater to healthcare professionals but also to individuals seeking to enhance their understanding of holistic wellness and thyroid health.

By sharing her wealth of knowledge and personal experiences, Dr. Wells aimed to demystify the complexities of hypothyroidism and empower people to make informed decisions about their well-being. She believed that by nurturing compassion and fostering a deeper understanding of the mind-body connection, individuals could unlock their innate healing potential and reclaim their vitality.

Moreover, Dr. Wells recognized the importance of building a strong community of like-minded individuals who shared her passion for holistic healing. She envisioned creating a platform where patients, practitioners, and advocates could connect, share their stories, and support one another on their journeys.

Through this community, she hoped to foster a sense of belonging and solidarity, reminding everyone that they were not alone in their struggles. By nurturing compassion and empathy, they could uplift and inspire one another, creating a ripple effect of positive change that would extend far beyond the clinic's walls.

As Dr. Wells gazed out the window, watching the world go by, she felt a deep sense of gratitude for the path that had led her to this moment. She knew that her work was not just about treating hypothyroidism; it was about nurturing compassion, empowering individuals, and creating a legacy of hope for generations to come.

With a renewed sense of determination, she picked up her pen and began to jot down her thoughts, envisioning a future where holistic wellness was not just a niche concept but a way of life embraced by all. It was a future where compassion and healing went hand in hand, and where the wisdom of nature was celebrated and revered.

12.4 Embracing Holistic Living

As Dr. Sarah Wells looked back on her journey, she couldn't help but feel a profound sense of gratitude for the path that had unfolded before her. What began as a seed of doubt had blossomed into a movement that transcended the boundaries of conventional medicine, embracing a holistic approach to wellness.

Through her unwavering dedication and the support of countless individuals who believed in her vision, Dr. Wells had not only transformed the lives of her patients but also inspired a paradigm shift in the way people viewed healthcare. The concept of holistic living had taken root, and its influence was spreading like wildfire.

At the heart of this movement was the understanding that true healing extended beyond the mere treatment of symptoms. It was a holistic approach that recognized the intricate interplay between the body, mind, and spirit. By addressing the root causes of imbalance and nurturing the body's innate ability to heal, Dr. Wells and her allies had paved the way for a more comprehensive and sustainable path to wellness.

The principles of holistic living were simple yet profound. They emphasized the importance of a balanced diet rich in whole, unprocessed foods, the incorporation of regular physical activity, and the cultivation of a positive mindset through practices like meditation and mindfulness. These pillars formed the foundation of a lifestyle that promoted overall well-being, rather than merely masking symptoms with synthetic medications.

As word of Dr. Wells's success spread, more and more individuals began to embrace the tenets of holistic living. They discovered the transformative power of making conscious choices about their diet, exercise routines, and stress management techniques. The results were nothing short of remarkable, with many reporting increased energy levels, improved mental clarity, and a newfound sense of vitality.

One of the most profound aspects of the holistic living movement was its ability to empower individuals to take an active role in their own healing journey. By understanding the interconnectedness of their physical, emotional, and spiritual well-being, people were able to make informed decisions and take responsibility for their health. This shift in mindset fostered a sense of agency and control, which in turn fueled a deeper commitment to sustainable lifestyle changes.

Dr. Wells's clinic became a beacon of hope and a hub for those seeking guidance on their path to holistic living. The once-skeptical medical community began to take notice, as the overwhelming success stories and scientific evidence supporting the efficacy of integrative approaches became impossible to ignore.

The clinic's doors were open to all, welcoming individuals from diverse backgrounds and walks of life. Here, patients found a safe haven where they could explore alternative therapies, receive personalized care, and connect with a community of like-minded individuals. The atmosphere was one of warmth, understanding, and unwavering support, fostering an environment conducive to healing on every level.

Beyond the clinic's walls, the ripples of change continued to spread. Dr. Wells and her team embarked on a mission to educate the public about the benefits of holistic living. They hosted workshops, seminars, and community events, sharing their knowledge and inspiring others to embrace a more balanced and fulfilling way of life.

The impact of this movement extended far beyond the realm of physical health. By encouraging individuals to cultivate a deeper connection with themselves, their loved ones, and the natural world around them, holistic living fostered a sense of purpose and belonging. It reminded people of the inherent beauty and resilience of the human spirit, and the power of embracing a lifestyle rooted in harmony and balance.

As the years passed, the legacy of Dr. Sarah Wells and her pioneering work in holistic wellness continued to grow. Her unwavering commitment to compassion, innovation, and the pursuit of true healing had ignited a fire that burned brightly, illuminating the path for countless individuals seeking a more fulfilling and sustainable way of life.

In the end, Dr. Wells's journey was not just about treating a condition; it was about empowering people to reclaim their health, their happiness, and their sense of wholeness. Through her dedication and the collective efforts of those who embraced her vision, the holistic living movement had become a beacon of hope, shining a light on the transformative power of embracing a life in harmony with nature and one's true self.

12.5 A Lasting Impact

As Dr. Sarah Wells stood on the podium, addressing the gathering of medical professionals and students, she couldn't help but reflect on the remarkable journey that had led her to this moment. The auditorium was filled with eager faces, all united by a shared desire to embrace a more holistic approach to healthcare.

"Today, we stand at the precipice of a new era in medicine," she began, her voice resonating with conviction. "An era where we recognize the profound wisdom of nature and the innate healing capabilities of the human body."

Dr. Wells paused, allowing her words to sink in. She knew that her message had the power to challenge long-held beliefs and ignite a paradigm shift in the way thyroid disorders, and indeed all health conditions, were perceived and treated.

"For too long, we have relied solely on synthetic medications and invasive procedures, often overlooking the profound healing potential that lies within the natural world," she continued. "But today, we have the opportunity to forge a new path – one that embraces the best of both conventional and alternative medicine."

As she spoke, Dr. Wells couldn't help but recall the countless patients whose lives had been transformed by her integrative approach. She remembered the joy on their faces as they regained their vitality, shed unwanted weight, and found emotional balance – all through the power of nature's gifts.

"The journey has been long and arduous, but the rewards have been immeasurable," she said, her eyes shining with determination. "We have witnessed firsthand the transformative effects of dietary changes, herbal remedies, acupuncture, and mindfulness practices. Lives have been forever changed, and hope has been restored."

Dr. Wells knew that her work had not only impacted the lives of her patients but had also inspired a new generation of healthcare professionals. She had ignited a spark within them, challenging them to question the status quo and seek out innovative solutions that honored the body's innate wisdom.

"Our clinic has become a beacon of hope, a sanctuary where individuals can find solace and healing," she said, her voice filled with pride. "But our mission extends far beyond these walls. We have a responsibility to share our knowledge and empower others to take control of their own well-being."

As she scanned the audience, Dr. Wells saw the faces of those who had once doubted her unconventional methods. Now, they sat with open minds and hearts, ready to embrace a new paradigm of healthcare that integrated the best of both worlds.

"The road ahead may be challenging, but together, we can overcome any obstacle," she declared. "We must continue to educate, inspire, and advocate for a more compassionate and holistic approach to healing. Only then can we truly create a lasting impact on the lives of those we serve."

With each word, Dr. Wells could feel the energy in the room shifting, as if a collective awakening was taking place. She knew that her message had struck a chord, igniting a fire within those present to become agents of change in their respective fields.

"Today, we stand united, a community of healers committed to nurturing the body, mind, and spirit," she said, her voice resonating with conviction. "Together, we will forge a legacy of hope – a legacy that transcends boundaries and inspires generations to come."

As the applause thundered through the auditorium, Dr. Wells felt a sense of profound gratitude wash over her. She had embarked on this journey with a seed of doubt, but now, she stood as a beacon of hope, guiding others towards a future where holistic healing was not just an alternative, but an integral part of modern healthcare.

In that moment, she knew that her work had transcended the realm of thyroid disorders and had become a catalyst for a broader movement – one that celebrated the profound wisdom of nature and the indomitable spirit of the human body. Her legacy would be one of compassion, innovation, and an unwavering commitment to empowering individuals to reclaim their well-being through the healing power of nature.

www.ingramcontent.com/pod-product-compliance
Lightning Source LLC
Chambersburg PA
CBHW061647250726
48659CB00004B/1407
* 9 7 9 8 3 2 0 6 4 9 8 0 1 *